T0214625

Precision Health and Artificial Intelligence

With Privacy, Ethics, Bias, Health Equity, Best Practices, and Case Studies

Arjun Panesar

Apress®

Precision Health and Artificial Intelligence: With Privacy, Ethics, Bias, Health Equity, Best Practices, and Case Studies

Arjun Panesar
DDM Health, University of Warwick,
Coventry, UK

ISBN-13 (pbk): 978-1-4842-9161-0   ISBN-13 (electronic): 978-1-4842-9162-7
https://doi.org/10.1007/978-1-4842-9162-7

Managing Director, Apress Media LLC: Welmoed Spahr
Acquisitions Editor: Celestin Suresh John
Development Editor: Laura Berendson
Coordinating Editor: Shrikant Vishwakarma
Copy Editor: Kim Wimpsett

Cover designed by eStudioCalamar

Cover image by Jason Leung on Unsplash (www.unsplash.com)

Distributed to the book trade worldwide by Apress Media, LLC, 1 New York Plaza, New York, NY 10004, U.S.A. Phone 1-800-SPRINGER, fax (201) 348-4505, e-mail orders-ny@springer-sbm.com, or visit www.springeronline.com. Apress Media, LLC is a California LLC and the sole member (owner) is Springer Science + Business Media Finance Inc (SSBM Finance Inc). SSBM Finance Inc is a **Delaware** corporation.

For information on translations, please e-mail booktranslations@springernature.com; for reprint, paperback, or audio rights, please e-mail bookpermissions@springernature.com.

Apress titles may be purchased in bulk for academic, corporate, or promotional use. eBook versions and licenses are also available for most titles. For more information, reference our Print and eBook Bulk Sales web page at www.apress.com/bulk-sales.

Any source code or other supplementary material referenced by the author in this book is available to readers on GitHub (https://github.com/Apress). For more detailed information, please visit www.apress.com/source-code.

Printed on acid-free paper

Dedicated to the infinite beauty of Kirpa, Ananta, Charlotte, and Akaal.

Table of Contents

About the Author

Arjun Panesar is the founding Chief Executive Officer and Head of AI at DDM Health, a multi-award-winning provider of digital therapeutics demonstrated to improve patient health outcomes, improve health equity, and unlock clinical efficiencies.

It was during the first year of his computing and artificial intelligence (AI) undergraduate master's degree at Imperial College, London, in 2002 that his grandfather, Anupam, was diagnosed with type 2 diabetes after emergency quadruple heart bypass surgery. Not knowing how to manage his lifestyle in a way that suited his cultural and social expectations, Anupam turned to Arjun for guidance on what to eat. It was at this point Arjun founded a global community for people with long-term health conditions.

Now with more than two decades of experience in healthcare and AI, Arjun leads the development of evidence-based digital health solutions that provide precision care to patients, health services, and governments across the globe. Arjun's work has received recognition from the BBC, Forbes, New Scientist, and The Times, and has been awarded an array of innovation, business, and technology awards. Most recently, the Gro Health app was rated the number-one digital health app in Europe by a health review body on behalf of the UK's National Health Service.

With more than a dozen published articles and three books, Arjun is a leading expert in AI, healthcare, and ethics. Arjun is an advisor to the Information School, University of Sheffield; Honorary Clinical Lecturer in Precision Medicine at Warwick Medical School, University of Warwick; and alumni fellow to the NHS Innovation Accelerator. He also has been recognized by Imperial College as an alumni leader for his contribution and impact to global health.

About the Technical Reviewer

Ashish Soni is an experienced AI/ML consultant and solutions architect. He has worked and solved business problems related to computer vision, natural language processing, machine learning, artificial intelligence, data science, statistical analysis, data mining, and cloud computing. Ashish holds a bachelor's of technology degree in chemical engineering from the Indian Institute of Technology, Bombay, India; a master's degree in economics; and a post-graduate diploma in applied statistics. He has worked across different industry areas such as finance, healthcare, education, sports, human resources, retail, and logistics automation. He currently works with a technology services company based out of Bangalore.

Acknowledgments

This book would not have been possible without the patience, tolerance, and encouragement of many people. A huge thank-you to the DDM Health team—particularly Amar, Harkrishan, and Dom—with whom many discussions on healthcare and the ethics of humankind took place. Thank you to Giverny for creating captivating imagery to complement the book; you are indeed the best graphic designer on the planet. Thank you to my partner, Charlotte, for listening to my meanderings. You continue to inspire me.

Thank you, Anish, for the meticulous detail and technical rigor to ensure the potential of this book was realized; and the fantastic team at Apress, particularly Mark and Celestin, for your encouragement, support, and motivation.

Introduction

Over the last decade, almost all industrial sectors have seen a technical revolution. Healthcare is no different, other than the fact that lives are at stake. While technological transformation within healthcare remains slow, the pandemic pushed everyone to engage in some form of digital technology. Unfortunately, the COVID lockdowns exposed a stark digital divide and highlighted the impact of the social determinants of health. However, the COVID recovery has spurred healthcare providers, catalyzed by start-ups, scale-ups, pharmaceutical companies, and academia, to replace the one-size-fits-all healthcare approach with one more focused on diversity to maximize health and well-being. Not before time, too. Healthcare providers face sicker people, mounting costs, stretched budgets, and staffing challenges.

Few remaining information gaps in healthcare require fusing the digital and analog worlds. Almost every human experience can now generate some form of data, and with this comes the growing ability to plot every aspect of the human experience, including health. As this data becomes part of the more comprehensive healthcare system, highly individualized healthcare and artificially intelligent algorithms become possible. Yet innovation is only one part of the problem. The ability for clinicians to implement technologies and for patients to benefit from them is a different theme altogether.

The more data, the more we can personalize and the more confident we can become in our predictions. Digitalization of healthcare is improving a broad range of outcomes but is still in its nascency. From the prevention of disease to rehabilitation and drug identification, with more data, more precise healthcare becomes possible. Treatment plans are individualized to accommodate better personal preferences concerning risk, medical interventions, or preferences. At a population level, health systems can use resources more efficiently, making them more effective and sustainable as communities age. But just like the advent of the Internet, it may be decades before healthcare can realize the benefits of precision health. Like people, AI and digital technologies can still get things wrong and have biases. Nevertheless, precision health remains centered on identifying and responding to each individual's health and well-being needs.

The connected world is weaving its way into our everyday, real-world lives. Before long, people will travel and control their own private data cloud as they use applications and other services. The aggregation of all individuals' data within the digital continuum, or the metaverse, enables deep digital phenotyping and digital twins composed of digital organs updated in real time by clinical diagnostics, sensors and wearables embedded, worn and ambient in the environment. Sensor technology is becoming increasingly pervasive and enables interaction without a keyboard or screen through voice, gesture, and brain interaction. All this data can be used to personalize our health, lifestyle, and behaviors to optimize our longevity and quality of life.

There are still notable challenges to overcome. Most health data is generated in silos, data remains unlinked, and people don't get access to it, never mind know how to use it. There are considerable variations in access and outcomes, and that's before the ethical and moral challenges involved.

The book provides a deep dive into the key topics within precision health. Starting with an introduction to the shift to value-based care, the book presents the five Ps of precision health, a framework for precision health, and explains the use of data and the digital phenotype. There is a section of the book dedicated to AI and machine learning in precision health, covering types of intelligence, computational approaches used in artificial intelligence, and the applicability of AI in areas such as drug discovery, patient care, and clinical decision support. Additionally, there is a section dedicated to the significant risks and ethical challenges posed by precision health systems. The book concludes with a selection of case studies exemplifying precision health technologies.

Audience

This book is a radically different alternative to books on precision health. It introduces healthcare professionals (nurses, physicians, practitioners, innovation officers), medical students, computing students, and data scientists to the use of data and AI in delivering precision healthcare and the critical considerations in its application without the need for endless code and mathematics.

This book is a valuable source for clinicians, healthcare workers, and researchers from diverse areas of the biomedical field who may or may not have a computational background and want to learn more about the innovative field of artificial intelligence for precision health.

CHAPTER 1

Introduction

Mobile technology has spread rapidly across the globe and is accomplishing more than just connecting people. The humble smartphone is responsible for changing the fundamentals of how we live—enabling users with a wealth of features including instant communication, Internet browsing, entertainment, games, productivity and location mapping.

As well as being magnitudes more powerful than the computers sitting onboard NASA's Perseverance Rover currently exploring Mars, smartphones are responsible for the growing datafication of our lives.[1] More than 8 in 10 people around the world own a smartphone. And each of these people carries their own private, unique data cloud.[2]

We generate data everywhere: our shopping habits, taxi journeys, music preferences, payment habits, social media interactions, DNA test results, food delivery orders, and messages all contribute to the 2.5 quintillion bytes of data we produce daily. In 2025, this is expected to

---

[1] The Perseverance rover runs on processors used in iMacs in the 1990s. [online] New Scientist. Available at: https://www.newscientist.com/article/2269403-the-perseverance-rover-runs-on-processors-used-in-imacs-in-the-1990s/.

[2] Statista (2022). Number of Smartphone Users Worldwide 2014-2020 | Statista. [online] Statista. Available at: https://www.statista.com/statistics/330695/number-of-smartphone-users-worldwide/.

© Arjun Panesar 2023
A. Panesar, *Precision Health and Artificial Intelligence*,
https://doi.org/10.1007/978-1-4842-9162-7_1

reach 463 exabytes (2^60 bytes).[3] Most aspects of our day-to-day lives are transferred into data and, from this, create an opportunity for making more optimal decisions.

People carry with them millions of data points that, to some degree of accuracy, can be used to define them. Smartphones, the Internet of Things, and the ubiquity of connectivity have enabled a moment-by-moment quantification of each person's individual state of being and human experience using data from digital devices that they use. As patients, we generate masses of data, collected within our medical records, smartphones, and other sources, which detail our prior health history, current health status, and, in a growing number of use cases, predisposition to future illness.

Growth in big data generation and its storage has been facilitated through scalable and affordable cloud services, and wherever there is data, there is artificial intelligence (AI). AI and machine learning have blossomed as disciplines, fueled by the data being generated and its availability. Autonomous vehicles, smart speakers, chatbots, and marketing are just some examples of how AI is used to empower humans to live in a more efficient and individualized way more than 60 years after the term was first defined. AI has famously beaten the greatest minds of chess and Go in competitions that humans have played for thousands of years.[4] With the introduction of AI capabilities, the ability to learn from data to make better decisions has never been more accessible.

When applied to healthcare, the mining of data of millions of patients enables machine learning to realize its potential and develop powerful AI algorithms to help predict disease and provide precise, individualized

---

[3] Bulao, J. (2022). How Much Data Is Created Every Day in 2022? [online] TechJury. Available at: https://techjury.net/blog/how-much-data-is-created-every-day/.

[4] 3 times AI beat human champions at their own game. [online] Alldus. Available at: https://alldus.com/blog/3-times-ai-beat-human-champions-at-their-own-game/.

treatment to each patient. The distinction between person and patient is critical as people's perspectives on technology and data sharing vary significantly depending on whether they are used for health or any other benefit.

Developing and interpreting the wealth of data produced by these technological and scientific innovations has already profoundly modified the scientific landscape. AI applications play an important role in fields like gene-editing CRISPR and drug discovery and AI-powered services such as monitoring health status and behavior change (or the art of suggesting actions to improve health and well-being). AI is demonstrating increasing impact and outcomes through the pervasive use of smartphones, biological data, and IoT.

The data now available, coupled with exponential progress in data storage, computational power, and connectivity, means precision health is no longer science fiction; it is a real-time reality.

From Personalized Medicine to Precision Health

Precision health is a medical paradigm that extends evidence-based practice and medicine. Precision health provides customized healthcare to the characteristics of each patient or group of patients rather than a one-size-fits-all model. Healthcare is not just delivered at the point of diagnosis but instead received from birth with tailored health and behavioral support.

Precision medicine and personalized medicine share many similarities. Personalized medicine is an older term generally referring to advanced -omics testing or biomarker discovery tools that are used to customize medical treatments based on an individual's unique biomarker profile.

Personalized medicine is entangled with precision health, with both terms now generally referring to the same thing. While genomic testing makes a person's DNA available and identifies gene single nucleotide polymorphisms (SNPs, the most frequent type of genetic variation among people), precision health accordingly facilitates personalized, evidenced-based health treatments. Precision health ensures that decisions, treatments, practices, and products are appropriate and optimal by using information about a person's genes, behaviors, and environment to provide tailored, patient-centered care. Another term used interchangeably with personalized medicine and precision health is 4P medicine, an acronym that denotes the principles of precision health.

This precise approach to medicine is not new. Healthcare professionals have been using this clinical approach since the time of Hippocrates. Yet never have humans had the power to predict illness and support health quite like today. A person's state of health is the collective product of their genetic makeup, medical history, microbiome, diet, lifestyle, and environment. Our body has 30 to 40 trillion cells, each with genetic codes compiled of billions of DNA base pairs; and our microbiome alone comprises more than 39 trillion microbes that are essential to our health and well-being. Each cell has an expression formed of subsets of genes that form complex relationships with health and well-being. Every person has a different genetic makeup and microbiome, needs a particular diet, and has a unique health status and personalized form of health, medicine and behaviors to obtain and maintain optimal health.

The hyper-personalization achievable from the patient genome and its falling cost, medical data from health records, wearable technology, and the health IoT, coupled with distributed hosting, has made it possible to move to personalized, real-time care.

Precision health is not only about enhanced risk profiling and population stratification, but it encompasses how that data is used to improve patient and population-level outcomes. Groups of patients, for example, may share common characteristics such as the risk of disease, similar to how one drug might not fit everyone's requirements.

Examples of precision health include the following:

- Biomarker testing to ensure the correct treatment is received. Blood transfusions require the blood transfused to match the patient's own blood type to ensure suitability and optimize the chances of recovery.

- The use of social media to track disease and communicate health information. Digital health was a critical tool in response to the COVID-19 pandemic and maintaining healthcare delivery during multiple global lockdowns. Data was used to record the spread and progression of the disease and to facilitate education, guidance, and support.

- Understanding medical options when there is a familial risk of disease to receive screening earlier or more often, take medicine or have surgery. For example, women with a mutation of the BRCA1 or BRCA2 gene are at higher risk of developing breast and ovarian cancer. Identifying such modifications earlier enables patients and healthcare teams to take action to prevent the disease or detect it earlier.

- Continuous glucose monitoring to optimize insulin dosing and behaviors. By using real-time data from glucose monitoring sensors, continuous glucose monitoring systems provide a range of benefits, including insulin dosing, encouraging positive health behaviors, preventing complications, and enabling the sharing of real-time health data with clinical teams. Importantly, granular blood glucose data indicates a user's state of health and behaviors more than traditional HbA1c tests that would typically occur every six months.

- Smartphone applications that provide behavioral change and chronic disease management support. Health applications monitor health and behaviors, encourage patients to adhere to treatments and behaviors, provide coaching, and prompt patients to attend appointments and screenings.

Precision health converges with Eastern medicine, mainly derived from Chinese and Indian cultures, which, like personalized medicine and systems medicine, considers human biological systems as a cohesive whole.[5] Eastern medicine views the human body as a holistic entity of harmonious organs and approaches health from this framework. Figure 1-1 demonstrates how precision health tools are used to provide care at all stages of a disease or, conversely, health.

[5] Sagner, M., McNeil, A., Puska, P., Auffray, C., Price, N.D., Hood, L., Lavie, C.J., Han, Z.G., Chen, Z., Brahmachari, S.K. and McEwen, B.S., 2017. The P4 health spectrum–a predictive, preventive, personalized and participatory continuum for promoting healthspan. Progress in cardiovascular diseases, 59(5), pp.506–521.

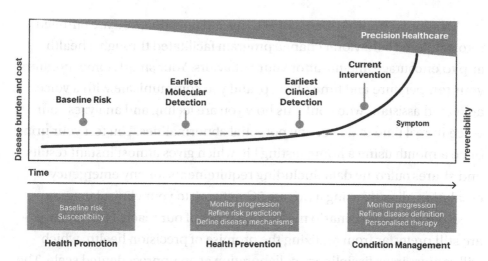

Figure 1-1. *Progression of disease on a precision health timeline*

Imagine now an ethically and morally utopian society where routine genomic screening tests occur once someone is born. You have your genome screened at birth, and there is a presentation of biomarkers that place you at higher risk of heart disease. Because of your familial and genetic risk of heart disease, you receive a smart patch that measures heart rate, blood pressure, and SpO2. As you grow older, you receive weekly cardiograms as part of a regular opt-in treatment program and smart patch replacements. All of your data is sent to a cloud-based ecosystem visible to your clinical team and next of kin. The next day, you receive a text message from your clinician, who is notified of your deteriorating health in real time to invite you for an appointment. You worry about what news you receive.

At your appointment, you are notified that there is the presence of particular electrolytes in your sweat, placing you at risk of heart failure. The activity data from your phone is assessed alongside your food diary app to conduct a risk assessment based on your health and recent behaviors. Your clinician gives you medicine that you take weekly that excretes a compound detected in your urine if symptoms of heart failure persist, and you are encouraged to improve your lifestyle.

To support improvements in activity and nutrition, you are enrolled into a tailored behavioral change program facilitated through a health app to encourage and monitor your behaviors. Your smart home monitors your temperature and time of sleep, and you communicate with a voice-activated assistant who confirms how you are feeling and analyzes your voice in real time to detect any potential abnormalities. You test your urine once a month using a home testing kit, which gives almost instant results and shares outcome data, including requirements for any emergency escalation, directly using a private 5G network to your clinical team.

No part of this scenario mentioned is out of our reach. However, we are still pretty far from realizing the promise of precision health, which will require interdisciplinary collaboration at an unprecedented scale. The reward? The benefits of precision health. Medicine, as currently practiced, is empirical, inadequately grounded in evidence, and dependent on the knowledge and experience of individual providers, which results in variable care with suboptimal outcomes.

Precision health enables patient-centered, individualized care tailored to the characteristics of patients at scale to provide patient-level and population-level health benefits. The goal is a unified approach to match a full range of promotion, prevention, diagnostic, and treatment interventions to fundamental and actionable determinants of health— to not just address symptoms but directly target genetic, biological, environmental, and social and behavioral determinants of health. Figure 1-2 provides a high-level overview of how precision health enables better health.

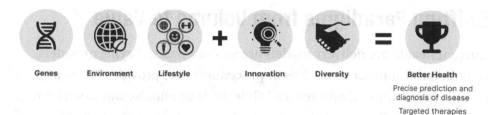

Figure 1-2. *Enabling better health with a precision health approach*

At its heart, precision health's objective is to prevent, predict, treat, and cure disease precisely.

That said, there are unprecedented challenges precision health poses that must be addressed to ensure precision health and AI safely and beneficially impact healthcare.

Why Precision Health? Why Now?

The world's population is living longer, unhealthier lives, and the global economy is in crisis.

Healthcare systems are stretched and turning to value-based and incentivized care as noncommunicable diseases (NCDs) such as obesity, cardiovascular disease, type 2 diabetes, and cancers become pandemics in their own right. The causes of these NCDs are rooted mainly in lifestyle and environmental factors that are challenging to modify, given the nature of modern environments, behaviors, and occupations. And that was before COVID-19.

Shifting Paradigms from Volume to Value

Current healthcare delivery models are volume-based. Paying providers based on the number of services or procedures they provide is known as *volume-based care* or *fee-for-service*. While this is an intuitive way to structure reimbursement, it does little to ensure systems are necessary or impactful.

Value-based care focuses on the patient. The quality of care is evaluated through the patient experience and outcomes, which continuously shapes how care is given and received. Through the integration of technology and medicine, value-based care has advanced a plethora of innovation that continues to improve lives. Value-based care is a refreshing perspective on healthcare.

Consider a hospital scenario, where instead of being compensated based on the number of patients appointments conducted, a hospital was compensated based on the number of patients in good health and the number of free beds available. Provider emphasis shifts from the time of hospital admission to forecasting future dangers and anticipating them with preventative strategies.

Value-based healthcare systems are changing the delivery of healthcare:

- From treating patient illness to managing health and well-being

- From one-size-fits-all to precision health solutions

- From a reactive healthcare system to a holistic, predictive healthcare system

- From length of life to quality of life over a lifetime

Given the financial strain healthcare systems face, value-based healthcare is a much-needed approach. The focus on outcomes requires quality management procedures including data generation, measurement, collection, and evaluation, which in turn facilitates improvement in care and efficiency.

As value-based healthcare systems grow, so too do the data they generate. Value-based care is facilitated through collaborative clinician-patient relationships in which data is shared or linked with consent so that care can be coordinated and reviewed across disciplines. Not only does this approach drive better healthcare, but it can reduce redundant care and its associated costs. Figure 1-3 shows how a connected health ecosystem could provide precision healthcare.

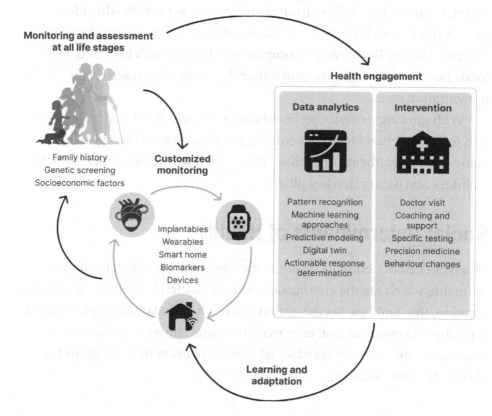

Figure 1-3. *How the patient cloud supports precision health*

In a value-based healthcare system, a patient at a greater risk of nonalcoholic fatty liver disease would be made aware of their risk as soon as possible and receive support to encourage positive health behaviors and self-manage their health. Help could come in the guise of cooking classes supported by a nutritionist to promote and encourage healthier behaviors. Regular diagnostic testing and monitoring would determine relevant biomarkers and their progress toward recommended targets.

Health, wearable, and electronic medical record data is shared between departments and organizations to develop a personalized nutrition and activity plan. Patients are supported to realize behavioral changes through digitally delivered programs that provide education, peer support, coaching, and resources such as recipes and on-demand exercise classes. By utilizing a companion-like approach to health, the focus becomes preventative care rather than providing reactive, on-presentation care.

With growing pressure on healthcare resources and lifestyle, behavior, and environmental factors accounting for 90 percent of disease risk, value-based healthcare underlines the role of lifestyle as medicine, making wellness and prevention key pillars.[6]

Social Determinants of Health

Precision health demands an understanding of the social determinants of health, which are the circumstances under which individuals are born, develop, live, and age. Socioeconomic position, education, neighborhood and physical environment, employment, social support, and access to healthcare are all examples of social determinants of health. Figure 1-4 shows the social determinants of health.

---

[6] Rappaport, S. M., & Smith, M. T. (2010). Environment and disease risks. Science, 330(6003), 460–461.

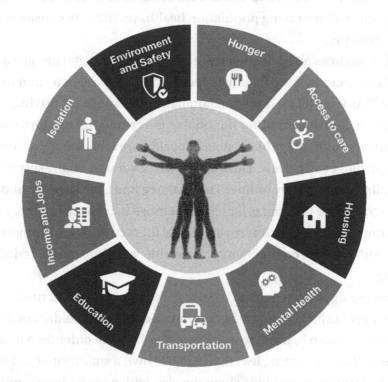

Figure 1-4. *Social determinants of health*

Research shows that the social determinants of health have a more significant impact on a person's health than medical intervention. Compared to medical services, the social determinants of health have twice the responsibility for health outcomes.[7]

Abundant research has shown that when it comes to patient-level care, gender, ethnicity, and neighborhood still have the most significant impact on accessing healthcare and achieving positive health outcomes. With greater reliance on digital tools, there is a risk of increasing health inequalities between those with skills and access to digital tools and those

---

[7] Mirkhani, R., & Ghorbani, F. (2021). Social Factors Affecting Chronic Diseases and Health. *International Journal of Medical Investigation, 10*(3), 1–15.

without. Precision health and social determinants of health entwine in their objective of improving population health, yet they are considered distinct concepts.

As they address all social determinants of health, digital literacy and Internet connectivity have been labeled the "super social determinants of health."[8] As you will no doubt be familiar, applications for driving, employment, housing, or other national or governmental support, each of which can affect an individual's state of health, are increasingly accessible online and often exclusively. During COVID lockdowns, many services were available exclusively online. The resource and time costs to empower a person to use the Internet is far less than those incurred by treating health conditions. Hence, improving digital literacy skills and empowering citizens with Internet connectivity can provide valuable tools to reduce disparities.

There are significant gaps in the use of the Internet within rural and socio-economically deprived communities alike and older adults. According to research, more than 60 percent of people older than 65 and 30 percent of those earning less than $30,000 own a smartphone, and many low-income households share devices, which poses access and privacy concerns for data purists.[9] Understanding the complexities of healthcare access in the communities that they serve can assist healthcare systems in implementing more inclusive policies to guarantee that no patient is left behind.

While it is unclear which social determinants of health best and most strongly relate to clinical and community health intervention, AI is seen as a communicator between the two constructs. A patient's social

---

[8] Herzog, L., Kellmeyer, P., & Wild, V. (2022). Digital behavioral technology, vulnerability and justice: towards an integrated approach. Review of Social Economy, 80(1), 7–28.

[9] Vangeepuram, N., Mayer, V., Fei, K., Hanlen-Rosado, E., Andrade, C., Wright, S., & Horowitz, C. (2018). Smartphone ownership and perspectives on health apps among a vulnerable population in East Harlem, New York. Mhealth, 4.

determinants can be merged with the patient's health-specific information and AI used to generate and map treatment protocols, with the sum of individual health closer to the nation's overall population health.

Addressing the social determinants of health is the primary focus for achieving equitable health access and outcomes. Health equity is realized when all people, regardless of their social position or environment, have the opportunity to attain their full health potential.

Why Diversity Is Essential Within Precision Health

My journey into precision health started in 2002 when I began an undergraduate master's degree in artificial intelligence at Imperial College, London.

At the end of my first semester, my grandfather, Anupam, was suddenly admitted to the hospital after suffering a heart attack and required an emergency quadruple heart bypass. Upon discharge, he was subsequently diagnosed with type 2 diabetes and instructed to follow a healthy, balanced diet. Not knowing how to manage his condition in a way that suited his Bengali-Indian lifestyle, my grandfather asked me for guidance on what to eat. I certainly had no idea, and neither did he, so we searched the Internet. What became immediately evident was the lack of content applicable to people like my grandfather, particularly to people from ethnic minority communities. He didn't need to be told about alternatives to sandwiches and breakfast cereals, but instead what to replace his roti, naan, and rice with. It was at this point I founded a global community for people with long-term health conditions. At that moment, a chance conversation about what my grandfather should eat to manage his newly acquired diagnosis turned into a passion for empowering people through data-driven, evidence-based digital health innovation. My role has provided unrivaled insight into a population of people with long-term health conditions, their families and caregivers, and the multitude of cultures and ethnicities that sit within this. As of 2022, ethnic minority communities are grossly misrepresented in healthcare. Today, as founding CEO at DDM Health, I am fortunate enough to lead a team that provides evidence-based precision digital therapeutics that care for more than 1.8 million people across seven countries in 19 native languages, existing to empower *everybody*.

Based on my own experiences and those of my family, I have been inspired to ensure under-represented communities are represented in, engaged in, and benefit from digital health. Using digital technology has provided an opportunity to engage people by personalizing a person's experience to their expectations, whether that is culture, language, social norms, or otherwise. By engaging and co-developing innovation with clinicians and patients, we have developed scalable, engaging, and effective solutions personalized for people of all heritage and not just those from ethnic minority communities.

Why is this important? Because achieving the goal of precision health for all requires the continued evaluation of what makes us different. Diversity is to be celebrated everywhere, and particularly within healthcare, as it serves as the means to a more inclusive, just, and effective healthcare system. It is crucial to understand disease through the context of human diversity, which isn't just about genetic heritage but also about how different people respond to illness and their environment. People's lived experiences are also data and expertise, and diversity enables us to engage and understand other cultures and worldviews. Not only does this overcome many biases—human bias, intelligence bias, machine bias, and data bias—but it also drives inspiration, innovation, and outcomes, self-realizing the goals of precision health. If digital health services are not provided equitably, bias becomes intrinsic, and quite frankly, that is a problem for everyone. Similarly, it is clear that healthcare services require an ethical and moral framework that it is our duty to be part of—to deliver, protect, and uphold.

Summary

Precision health holds tremendous promise for improving all aspects of healthcare. Some of these benefits have already been realized in the form of clinical decision tools, digital therapeutics, and -omics technologies, but a connected ecosystem is many decades away. Precise, tailored healthcare, from pediatrics to palliative, will be realized only once technologies, datasets, and communications are available ubiquitously. Until then, precision health acts in silos and will empower selected communities. Thus, precision health requires active responsibility and leadership from all stakeholders to ensure its benefits are realized by everyone.

CHAPTER 2

What Is Precision Health?

Precision health is a holistic healthcare approach that integrates numerous biological data points, including longitudinal molecular, cellular, and phenotypic biomarkers and individual genome sequences. Excluding the role of genetics, research shows four broad factors influence our health.[1]

- Social and economic environment: 40 percent

- Health behaviors: 30 percent

- Clinical care: 20 percent

- Physical environment: 10 percent

While the weightings may differ between individuals, the concept of precision health is to optimize all aspects of health through a new era of human health, which enables us to do the following:

- **Predict** the risk of disease when it can be controlled and reversed effectively.

---

[1] Evans, R. G., Barer, M. L., & Marmor, T. R. (Eds.). (1994). Why are some people healthy and others not?: The determinants of the health of populations. Transaction Publishers.

- **Prevent** disease development and their associated risk factors by implementing effective, evidence-based interventions at all levels.

- Provide care with the **participation** of the patient.

- Provide **personalized** treatments through more specific definitions of disease phenotypes that encourage the selection of optimal therapies and new biochemical targets for interventions.

- Provide a precision approach to **population** health. Diverting the typically reactive emphasis of medicine to that of a proactive, preventative ecosystem that focuses on health before disease enhances the concept of wellness in disease-free individuals and those with long-term conditions alike.

On average, patients typically interact with the healthcare system for 10 hours per year.[2] Attempts to make healthcare more predictive, preventive, personalized, participatory, and for the benefit of individuals and populations (described as P5 healthcare, as shown in Figure 2-1) will significantly improve health and well-being across the health continuum and is a new era for human health.

---

[2] www.cdc.gov. (2022). Exposome and Exposomics | NIOSH | CDC. [online] Available at: https://www.cdc.gov/niosh/topics/exposome/.

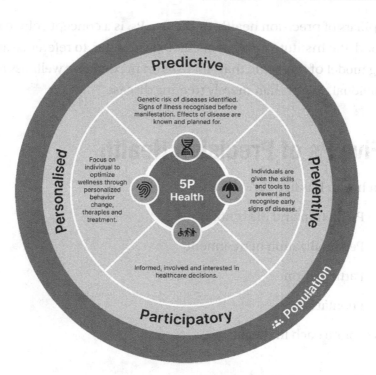

Figure 2-1. *Five Ps of precision health*

The precision health era started when scientists sequenced 92 percent of the human genome in 2003.[3] Digital health launched as a concept in 2007 when the first health and wellness apps were founded.[4] Alongside this, the idea of grid or cloud computing took huge strides forward with the launch of Amazon Web Service (AWS) and Elastic Compute Cloud (EC2) technology, which decoupled software development from server hosting and administration for the first time.

---

[3] National Institutes of Health (NIH). (2022). First complete sequence of a human genome. [online] Available at: https://www.nih.gov/news-events/nih-research-matters/first-complete-sequence-human-genome.

[4] Ventola, C.L., 2014. Mobile devices and apps for health care professionals: uses and benefits. Pharmacy and Therapeutics, 39(5), p.356.

The pillars of precision health, or the five Ps, is a concept coined by Leroy Hood, the Institute for Systems Biology founder, to reference an emerging model of medicine that "focuses on maximizing wellness for each individual, rather than merely treating disease."

The Five Ps of Precision Health

Precision health has five core pillars.

- Prediction and prevention

- Personalization of treatment

- Participation

- Population

Let's explore each in detail.

Prediction and Prevention

It is feasible that, in the future, requiring medical intervention may increasingly be seen as a failure of prevention. Precision prevention enables an improved overall state of health and better use of healthcare resources through several mechanisms: genetic testing, consumer technologies, and data analytics.

Rather than relying on familial history alone, the use of "-omics" technologies provides detailed data about an individual's genetic makeup, biochemical processes, and risk of particular diseases.[5]

Genetic screening tests are available to determine the risk of inherited breast and ovarian cancer syndrome, lynch syndrome, hereditary colon

---

[5] Karczewski, K.J. and Snyder, M.P., 2018. Integrative omics for health and disease. Nature Reviews Genetics, 19(5), pp.299–310.

and uterine cancers, and familial hypercholesterolemia inherited high cholesterol, among others. Learning about potential health risks enables clinicians and patients to follow personalized treatments and support behavioral change and clinical guidelines to address identified risks.

These are -omics technologies:

- *Genomics*: Genes, information on genetic predisposition

- *Transcriptomics*: RNA, information gene activity/ expression

- *Proteomics*: Proteins, information on key molecules that control cell biology

- *Metabolomics*: Cellular metabolites, information on enzymatic activities, and biochemistry of cells

The potential of precision prevention is vast, limited only by the data and computational power available.

As "multi-omics" data is embedded within clinical practice and the Internet of Everything is realized through connecting more extensive networks of people, processes, data, and things, a more comprehensive description of biological systems and health states is understood. Monitoring health states will enable prevention to move from a one-disease, one-test approach to risk prediction within new therapeutic areas. Integrating genomics, phenomics, and behavioral data driven by intelligent, connected devices and communications provides a rich mining dataset and enables a new age of disease prediction and prevention.

A significant challenge is integrating data in the context of the complexities of biological networks and constructing models of health and wellness that are both predictive and actionable, or, in other words, beneficial to both patients and clinicians.

The complexity of integrating data is a challenge best demonstrated in representing the predictive factors of obesity, which are multifaceted.

- Genetic factors such as genes and gene expression

- Individual lifestyle factors, such as dietary intake, exercise habits, TV viewing patterns, and income

- Environmental factors, such as the distance from grocery stores, walking environment, and food advertising

- School-related factors such as the availability of sugary beverages, distance to fast-food outlets, and school health education

- Industry factors such as portion-size norms in restaurants and packaged foods; state policies and regulation of food marketing

- National food distribution programs and support for various agricultural products

- Life-course factors such as the history of breastfeeding, maternal health, and parental obesity[6]

Genetic testing at birth will enable humans to optimize their lives by living in a way to prevent disease and detect their disposition to any particular disease based on available data. Data analysis is required to drive meaningful outcomes and provide optimal engagement and behavioral change opportunities. In other words, precision health enables data-driven medicine from birth to death.

---

[6] Khoury, M. J., Gwinn, M., Glasgow, R. E., & Kramer, B. S. (2012). A population perspective on how personalized medicine can improve health. American journal of preventive medicine, 42(6), 639.

Digital phenotyping, or the use of smart devices to collect data from available sensors that are received through human interaction with physical hardware and software to infer individual behaviors, will become more specific only as big datasets turn into vast datasets. Simple social media behaviors have already been linked to poor mental health, so using the digital phenotype to understand health and wellness in the form of digital indications derived from available data stands to unlock a treasure trove of potential.[7]

Personalization of Treatment

Personalized medicine and health programs can enable tailored treatments, reduce disease burden, improve quality of life, increase survival rates, and reduce the cost of care. Much of health is already personalized to characteristics, including age and gender. However, with genetic, environmental, biomedical, and lifestyle data, healthcare will develop a better understanding of the genome, interventions, and treatments.

For instance, most drugs are developed through clinical trials and intended for patients classified by disease group, assuming that the groups will have similar responses to treatment.[8] Moving from the conventional classification of diseases to using biomarkers to assist in stratifying types and subtypes of distinct conditions will enable better-personalized therapies through clinical research.

Personalizing preventative treatment and healthcare according to patient preferences such as preferred language, faith, and accessibility needs will significantly improve engagement and long-term outcomes

---

[7] Abi-Jaoude, E., Naylor, K. T., & Pignatiello, A. (2020). Smartphones, social media use and youth mental health. Cmaj, 192(6), E136–E141.

[8] Huang, L. K., Chao, S. P., & Hu, C. J. (2020). Clinical trials of new drugs for Alzheimer disease. Journal of biomedical science, 27(1), 1–13.

for many people. Personalization also supports the reduction of health inequalities by addressing some of the vital inertia to engaging with healthcare. From providing prescription labels in the native language to delivering health programs tailored to accessibility needs, personalization can take place across the healthcare spectrum to improve engagement and health outcomes.

Obesity is a significant risk factor for noncommunicable diseases and a cause of global economic burden. With value-based healthcare's approach to wellness, diet and nutrition are vital areas where populations can realize the impact of precision personalization. The field of nutrigenomics focuses on providing an optimal diet for each individual based on genotype supported through a tailored eating plan. Patients can use precision behavioral change tools to receive encouragement and maintain adherence. Figure 2-2 gives an indication of how individual-level data can be used to enhance the health of people.

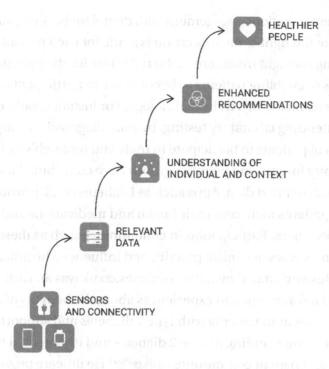

Figure 2-2. *Enhancing the health of people through understanding the individual*

Participation

Participation changes the role of the patient from being a passive recipient of care to a responsible, active, and well-informed patient at the center of their care. Patients (or carers where patients are unable to provide consent) are involved in all aspects of their care, including supported decision-making, self-monitoring, self-management of health, goal-setting, and behavioral change. Participation is a whole-systems approach to engage patients and, more important, support clinicians in engaging patients within their health. Clinician apathy has been long demonstrated to be a key component in patient engagement with digital tools.[9] Precision health aims to ensure the right clinical decision is made for each patient rather than providing the right treatment at the right time for the right patient.

Examples of enabling patients to become active participants in their care are primarily driven by technology. For instance, rather than repeatedly attending laboratory testing, by-mail diagnostic testing allows wider groups of patients to participate in trials and research studies.

Community forums and member groups have contributed a significant amount of unstructured data. Apps such as Diabetes.co.uk provide a platform for patients to discuss their health and medications and share personal experiences. Participation in communities such as these has encouraged new ways of clinical practice and influenced healthcare paradigms. Research has shown that Diabetes.co.uk was an early platform that collected information and experiences about the benefits of a low carbohydrate diet from patients with type 2 diabetes and supported a change in the understanding of type 2 diabetes and its potential treatments with clinical and patient communities alike.[10, 11] Healthcare providers can use growing data pools to define and refine the precision health experience.

A key aspect of digital participation is the mode of access. Enabling multiplatform participation ensures maximum accessibility for diverse and seldom-heard communities. For example, 60 percent of people older than 65 in the UK do not own a smartphone, meaning digital technologies

---

[9] Scott, E., Shehata, M., Panesar, A., Summers, C. and Dale, J., 2022. The Low Carb Program for people with type 2 diabetes and pre-diabetes: a mixed methods feasibility study of signposting from general practice. BJGP open, 6(1).

[10] Wu, P.F. and Bernardi, R., 2020. Community attachment and emotional well-being: an empirical study of an online community for people with diabetes. Information Technology & People.

[11] Saslow, L. R., Summers, C., Aikens, J. E., & Unwin, D. J. (2018). Outcomes of a digitally delivered low-carbohydrate type 2 diabetes self-management program: 1-year results of a single-arm longitudinal study. JMIR diabetes, 3(3), e9333.

and health programs require multimodal access and digital exclusion support to ensure access and equity. [12]

Notwithstanding, smart homes have the potential to move whole communities out of digital exclusion and support smart living, healthy aging, and longevity. Smart homes are adequate for home healthcare delivery as technologies can enable cost improvements and improve independence. It's not long before a dwelling is controlled through a virtual assistant operating the home's alarm clock, temperature, and solar panels and receiving package deliveries by drone. People's habits and behaviors are increasingly tracked to provide data that allows intelligent insights. Bluetooth-enabled water bottles, for instance, can confirm how much hydration has been received by an older person. As homes become more competent and cheaper to furnish with IoT devices, healthcare will naturally involve participants in day-to-day living, supporting the optimization of moment-by-moment wellness.

Population

The fifth P, the population perspective, is required to fulfill the notion of precision health. With good reason: precision health enables population health to realize its aim of empowering all without disparity. A population perspective integrates precision health into the ecologic model of health. The approach applies the principles of population screening to preventive medicine and uses evidence-based practice to personalize medicine delivery. Treatment is then appropriately delivered across the three core functions of public health: health promotion, prevention of ill health, and health protection.

Population health stands to improve by applying complementary individual and public health approaches to healthcare and disease prevention. However, this requires focusing on health's social and

---

[12] Serafino, P. (2019). Exploring the UK's digital divide. Office for National Statistics.

environmental determinants to address health inequalities. Balanced strategies that implement individual and population-level interventions can maximize health benefits, minimize harm, and avoid unnecessary healthcare costs. With growing awareness of the nuances of population-level data, bias, and support in engaging harder-to-reach communities, the potential benefits of five P care are limited only by the data available.

Considerations of Precision Health

While precision health holds great promise, there are several considerations to be aware of.

Cost

The cost of precision health is twofold: money and time. While genome sequencing and genetic testing costs are decreasing, the still-prohibitive cost of these technologies is a critical barrier to realizing precision health.[13] The probability of disease complications also affects the cost-effectiveness of precision health interventions. For instance, a patient with late-stage pancreatic cancer may benefit from a precision health intervention. However, the cost-effectiveness would be lower as the potential benefit, and health outcomes that the patient can realize are lower. It is feasible that healthcare providers will conduct testing at birth and earlier stages of the disease pathway to make genetic testing cost-effective and facilitate early-stage treatments.

---

[13] Christofyllakis, K., Bittenbring, J. T., Thurner, L., Ahlgrimm, M., Stilgenbauer, S., Bewarder, M., & Kaddu-Mulindwa, D. (2022). Cost-effectiveness of precision cancer medicine-current challenges in the use of next generation sequencing for comprehensive tumour genomic profiling and the role of clinical utility frameworks. Molecular and Clinical Oncology, 16(1), 1-4.

Clinicians delivering precision health and patients receiving precision care must understand how to use their respective technologies. All clinical stakeholders require training on new technologies, procedures, and policies to deliver precision healthcare. Similarly, patients receiving care through digital apps and devices need to understand how to use the technologies involved in their care. Healthcare providers would expect both types of training from the developers of the precision health tool. Additional software licenses and devices also represent pertinent, often unconsidered costs.

The benefits of precision healthcare commercialization include pricing that is transparent and nonprohibitive. The misguided incentives of volume-based care are replaced with outcomes-based models that re-incentivize providers. For instance, digital health companies such as DDM Health utilize outcomes-based models in large-scale deployments of precision health self-management tools.[14] The model is nonprohibitive and enables scalable models that realize the tenets of value-based care.

Genes Are Just the Beginning

Healthcare tailored to a patient's genetic profile vastly improves health outcomes in terms of pharmacogenomics, day-to-day behavioral change, and living well. Genetic testing at birth can undoubtedly support these moment-by-moment healthcare optimizations. However, the potential consequences of genetic testing, including discrimination, distress, and unintended consequences, are largely unexplored.

The genomics era of healthcare urgently needs a precision public health ethics framework that integrates the critical moral commitments and ethical requirements of precision medicine and traditional public health.

---

[14] NHS Innovation Accelerator. No funding? Maybe it's worth a risk. [online] Available at: https://nhsaccelerator.com/insight/no-funding-take-a-risk.

Health Equality

Medical care received by a patient in treating a disease plays a minor role in someone's overall health outcomes. Precision healthcare, which lends itself to digital tools, enables more accessible solutions that improve accessibility to communities that are typically hard to reach. While it can be complex, co-designing technologies with service providers and service users is crucial to mitigate inequalities. Apps such as Gro Health provide patient-centered or citizen-centered, cardiometabolic, and mental health interventions in 19 languages, demonstrating higher acceptance from ethnic minority communities compared to Caucasian counterparts.[15]

Digital exclusion is an eminent topic in precision healthcare. People who are digitally excluded may lack the skills, confidence, and motivation to use digital tools, along with not having access to suitable equipment and connectivity. Digital exclusion may occur for many reasons, which stakeholders can identify through analysis of the social determinants of health. While inequalities are mitigated for people with visual impairments, hearing impairments, accessibility difficulties, and non-English-speaking populations, digitally excluded populations represent a tenth of the population that often has more costly medical needs.[16] Although this population is decreasing slowly, the COVID pandemic pushed almost everybody online, and new technologies, such as private

---

[15] Abdelhameed, F., Pearson, E., Hanson, P., Barber, T., Panesar, A., & Summers, C. (2022, May). Health outcomes following engagement with a digital health tool GroHealth app amongst people with type 2 diabetes. In Endocrine Abstracts (Vol. 81). Bioscientifica.

[16] Good Things Foundation. The digital divide. [online] Available at: https://www.goodthingsfoundation.org/the-digital-divide/.

5G networks, enable connected device use in rural areas. In many rural areas, initiatives are focused on embedding pervasive communications within communities and layering health and social care services on top of this.[17]

Unfulfilled Power of Data

The distributed nature of clinical systems means that patient data is fragmented, and there is little coordination between healthcare providers. For instance, patients moving from border localities often have to re-register with clinical services that do not have access to the same patient information. The unification of patient data will take some time to accomplish. Nevertheless, data linkages are seeing positive progress with technologies such as FIHR, API, and SSO that facilitate protocols and standards for data sharing, storage, and communication.

Enabling a patient to store and control their own data (that is, any piece of data that is about or refers to a patient) is the pinnacle of data governance in precision health, putting the patient in control and taking the onus away from healthcare providers. Precision health continuously tracks data and actively applies it to the current moment to detect disease earlier, further personalize treatment, and prevent health deterioration. Availability and understanding of analytics to use the insights generated by the data collected will further facilitate service optimization and efficiencies.

While data linkages predominantly focus on structured medical data sources, unstructured data such as emails, text messages, WhatsApp messages, audio notes, Facebook posts, Twitter tweets, and other social

---

[17] The Scotsman. How digital technology is boosting healthcare. [online] Available at: https://www.scotsman.com/news/opinion/columnists/how-digital-technology-is-boosting-healthcare-arjun-panesar-3789087.

media posts are a treasure trove of information and insight that have been demonstrated to be predictors of health status but are not currently used within healthcare.[18]

Engagement

Precision health works only if both clinicians and patients are engaged. While the relationship between clinician and patient has become more collaborative and patient-centered, clinician engagement remains crucial. Research shows that clinician apathy can affect patient engagement in health apps.

Awareness is a critical piece regarding the benefits of digital and precision health. Awareness serves not only the purpose of showcasing technologies and their benefits but also the use of data and its potential implications. Training clinical teams and patients to use digital technology is required to prevent inadequate or incorrect treatments and understand the barriers to accessing support for digitally excluded patients, which is vital to provide democratic, accessible services.

A core tenet of precision health and value-based healthcare is patient-centered care, which ultimately serves the patient only if they engage. Engagement is akin to how a medication works if patients adhere to their medication regime. Digitally delivered behavioral change support has been demonstrated to actively engage and maintain patients in positive habits and behaviors such as healthier eating, more activity, better sleep,

[18] Ellington, M., Connelly, J., Clayton, P., Lorenzo, C. Y., Collazo-Velazquez, C., Trak-Fellermeier, M. A., & Palacios, C. (2022). Use of Facebook, Instagram, and twitter for recruiting healthy participants in nutrition-, physical activity-, or obesity-related studies: a systematic review. The American Journal of Clinical Nutrition, 115(2), 514-533.

and improved mental health.[19, 20] A mobile health app co-developed by a clinical hospital obesity team and its patients to provide behavioral change support for patients diagnosed with severe and morbid obesity showed significant improvements in self-reported health status after 12 weeks of use. There is a massive demand for health and well-being solutions that demonstrate clinical efficacy. However, long-term engagement has been shown only in a few applications and requires further long-term research.

High Touch Means High Tech

Technology and attention are required to make precision healthcare a reality. High-touch, high-intensity healthcare has been shown to improve health outcomes and lower costs. The use of apps, devices, and wearables to collect data and provide behavioral support and real-time clinical and patient decision support mechanisms is well demonstrated. A recent peer-reviewed study showed a digital health app used by patients with severe obesity within a hospital-based obesity service during COVID provided superior care compared to the hospital's traditional face-to-face dietetic supervision when delivered alongside remote appointments. The cost of digital interventions is far less than conventional face-to-face care, enabling greater scales of impact and economy.[21]

---

[19] Summers, C., Wu, P. and Taylor, A.J., 2021. Supporting Mental Health During the COVID-19 Pandemic Using a Digital Behavior Change Intervention: An Open-Label, Single-Arm, Pre-Post Intervention Study. JMIR Formative Research, 5(10), p.e31273.

[20] Summers, C. and Curtis, K., 2020. Novel Digital architecture of a "Low Carb Program" for initiating and maintaining long-term sustainable health-promoting behavior change in patients with type 2 diabetes. JMIR diabetes, 5(1), p.e15030.

[21] Hanson, P., Summers, C., Panesar, A., Oduro-Donkor, D., Lange, M., Menon, V. and Barber, T.M., 2021. Low Carb Program Health App Within a Hospital-Based Obesity Setting: Observational Service Evaluation. JMIR Formative Research, 5(9), p.e29110.

A high-touch, high-tech approach utilizes advances in technology and data to unlock information about healthcare efforts within populations, allowing for better targeting of those efforts.

Phenomics

Phenomics refers to the changes in an organism that result in phenotype variations during its life span, or, in other words, a set of phenotypes on a genome-wide scale that broadly deals with an organism's physical and biochemical traits. A personalized therapeutic strategy could theoretically suit someone's biological or genetic phenotype. Still, it could fail because of their stress level, dietary habits, working or living environment, or cultural background.

Deep digital phenotyping involves the combination of deep phenotyping (the precise and comprehensive analysis of phenotypic abnormalities in which the individual components of the phenotype are observed and described) and digital phenotyping (the real-time quantification of the particular human phenotype using real-world data from digital devices). Deep digital phenotyping achieves the ultimate goal of precision health: to match one individual, given their unique profile, with their best medical, therapeutic, and preventive strategy to maintain an optimal state of wellness, regardless of health status.

Digital Transformation

Precision health is an ambitious healthcare approach that dynamically connects research and practice, medicine, population, and public health. Coordinated efforts in developing clinician digital literacy standards, training, upskilling, and confidence are required to realize the approach.

However, most clinicians are already overburdened and experiencing burnout, fueled by the COVID pandemic and recovery.[22] One would theorize that digital transformation is best suited to a dedicated team that augments existing clinical deliveries rather than adding additional burden to already busy and overworked clinicians whose area of expertise is unlikely in the implementation of digital health solutions. A dedicated team could comprise nonclinical specialists whose sole activities are to augment the digital transformation ambitions. The paradigm is similar to that seen in digital health, where digital care practices supplement traditional care rather than replace it.

Multidisciplinary digital transformation teams allow stakeholders to focus on their key competencies, reduce unnecessary burdens, and provide a collaborative approach to digital health implementation.

With life expectancy declining, precision health facilitates new ways of living well, moving from a reactive to a proactive healthcare model. Table 2-1 highlights core changes in the shift to a proactive precision health approach.

[22] Palamara, K. and Sinsky, C., 2022, January. Four key questions leaders can ask to support clinicians during the COVID-19 pandemic recovery phase. In Mayo Clinic Proceedings (Vol. 97, No. 1, pp. 22-5). Elsevier.

Table 2-1. *Key Changes in the Shift from a Reactive to a Proactive Precision Health Approach*

Reactive Medicine	Precision Medicine
Symptoms-based response	Proactive and preventative, pre-symptom biomarker response
Disease management	Lifestyle health management
Few measurements	Multi-measurement, holistic
Organ- and disease-centric	Systems-centric
Symptom-focused therapy	Disease mechanism–focused therapy and intervention
Clinician led	Collaborative relationship

As the adoption of precision health technologies rises, so too will improvements in health outcomes, costs, and understanding.

Applying Precision Health: The P5H Precision Healthcare Continuum

The focus of healthcare in a precision health continuum is wellness, an optimal state of health, which acts as a core tenet in catalyzing healthcare's shift from volume-based to value-based care. [23]

Figure 2-3 illustrates the P5 healthcare continuum (P5H) model, adapted from the P4H model proposed by Sagner et al. to provide a population-level approach.[24]

---

[23] Vogt, H., Hofmann, B. and Getz, L., 2016. The new holism: P4 systems medicine and the medicalization of health and life itself. Medicine, Health Care and Philosophy, 19(2), pp.307–323.

[24] Sagner, M., McNeil, A., Puska, P., Auffray, C., Price, N.D., Hood, L., Lavie, C.J., Han, Z.G., Chen, Z., Brahmachari, S.K. and McEwen, B.S., 2017. The P4 health spectrum—a predictive, preventive, personalized and participatory continuum for promoting healthspan. Progress in cardiovascular diseases, 59(5), pp.506–521.

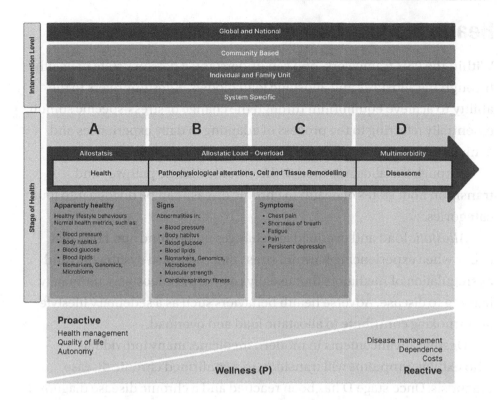

Figure 2-3. *P5 healthcare continuum (P5H) model that seeks to optimize wellness (P)*

The two central components of the P5H continuum consist of health stage and intervention level, with the primary objective of optimizing patient well-being or wellness.

The P5H framework focuses on promoting wellness, detecting and reversing disease transitions, and maintaining an optimal state of wellness.

Health Stages

Within the P5H framework, one can understand a person's state of health through the allostasis and allostatic load models. *Allostasis* refers to the ability to achieve equilibrium through the change of stress-specific stimuli, essentially referring to the process of adapting to daily experiences and achieving homeostasis through change.

Through the allostasis model, the chronic disease pathway and transition from states of health to chronic disease can be divided into four categories.

Allostatic load and overload are changes in the mind and body that occur when experiencing harmful stress that can cause dysfunction and dysregulation of mediators that usually promote homeostasis, ultimately leading to disease. Adverse health behaviors such as a sedentary lifestyle and smoking contribute to allostatic load and overload.

Despite advancements in modern medicine, many individuals who exhibit symptoms will transition to a confirmed chronic disease diagnosis. Once stage D has been reached and a chronic disease diagnosis confirmed, there is usually some degree of permanent physiologic damage or dysfunction. For example, a heart attack, stroke, cancer, or other long-term diseases will leave permanent damage and dysfunctions that typically require lifelong treatment and self-management. However, this is not true of all conditions, such as type 2 diabetes, which have been successfully reversed or placed into remission after significant long-term dysfunction.

Stage A

Stage A refers to a healthy individual exhibiting healthy lifestyle characteristics such as regular physical activity, no smoking, a nutritious diet, and no alcohol misuse, and possessing key health biomarkers such as blood glucose, blood pressure, and blood lipids within normal range.

As molecular assessments become available for a broader population, the definition and characterization of apparent health in stage A will become more precise and detailed.

Moving from allostasis to a pre-chronic disease state (stage B) is often unnoticed until the signs of chronic disease risk become imminent.

Through the accumulation of stressors or allostatic load, a person moves from stage A to stage B. The -omics technologies are helpful in stage A to determine genetic disposition to a disease before signs of allostatic load and clinical biomarkers exhibit.

Stage B

Stressors manifest as noticeable signs or biological expressions of disease. Diagnostic testing can detect early disease and biological dysfunction indicators, but the individual is often unaware of them. Examples include elevated blood glucose levels (i.e., prediabetes), hypertension, and high blood cholesterol. Chronic inflammation is an important sign of disease risk. In this approach, lifestyle habits such as engaging in below-normal levels of exercise and excess body weight would be considered signs of increased chronic disease risk.

Patients at stage B can benefit from preventive interventions to eliminate stressors and return an individual to stage A. In the absence of this, a patient's health will increasingly worsen.

Stage C

Healthcare delivered today is typically initiated when patients present with disease symptoms, or stage C, frequently treating the symptoms of disease rather than its underlying causes and dysfunction-causing mechanisms. Volume-based healthcare perpetuates this reactive cycle, where symptoms typically worsen without direct intervention until the allostatic overload reaches a threshold and chronic disease is diagnosed.

Stage D

At stage D, chronic disease is diagnosed, and treatment ensues. Traditional healthcare is delivered and uptitrated with pharmacotherapy, surgery, behavioral change, and other interventions used to manage chronic disease. Even at this stage of health, patients in a precision health model can improve their prognosis, clinical status, and quality of life. Environmental and behavioral factors are modifiable risks that directly impact wellness.[25]

Optimization Across Stages

The function of the precision health continuum is to optimize the state of wellness, with an individual even having the potential to reverse their state of health. Stages A to D are dynamic and omnidirectional, directly affected by genetics, health, physical and social environment, and behaviors.

While not replicable in all diseases, type 2 diabetes is an example of a condition once considered chronic and progressive that is now regarded as reversible. Lifestyle and behavioral interventions at stages B, C, and D have demonstrated reversal of prediabetes (a precursor to type 2 diabetes) and type 2 diabetes to normoglycemic levels. A digital health app, Low Carb Program, received global attention for reversing type 2 diabetes in an elderly patient diagnosed with the condition for more than 23 years. The digital platform, which provides patients with structured diabetes education and behavioral change support to adopt a nutritious diet and increase physical activity, supported a 67-year-old male to reverse his

---

[25] Kubzansky, L.D., Huffman, J.C., Boehm, J.K., Hernandez, R., Kim, E.S., Koga, H.K., Feig, E.H., Lloyd-Jones, D.M., Seligman, M.E. and Labarthe, D.R., 2018. Positive psychological well-being and cardiovascular disease: JACC health promotion series. Journal of the American College of Cardiology, 72(12), pp.1382–1396.

condition in 12 weeks.[26] The correct clinical decision can be made for any patient to optimize their state of well-being at any stage of the P5H framework.

Intervention Levels

There are four levels of intervention in the P5H continuum.

Level 1

Level 1 interventions are delivered globally or nationally, also understood as public health. The World Health Organization is a leading example of an organization with a public health focus, working at a national level to improve health understanding and engagement. Governments and national organizations have their own health themes based on local needs that ultimately seek to optimize the health of their respective populations and prevent chronic disease.

Level 2

Local communities often share similar needs and behaviors. An intervention at level 2 creates healthy environments and makes nutritious and affordable food readily available to individuals in local communities. Physical activity and mental well-being opportunities are provided, smoke and pollution are kept to a minimum, information and resources are provided on maintaining health and preventing chronic diseases, and healthy lifestyle behaviors are encouraged in healthcare systems. Interventions can be promoted wherever individuals live, work, or engage with public services such as schools.

---

[26] Weston, A. (2022). Man loses almost three stone in 12 weeks and reverses diabetes. [online] Liverpool Echo. Available at: https://www.liverpoolecho.co.uk/news/liverpool-news/man-loses-almost-three-stone-23192429.

Level 3

Interventions are successful only if an individual engages or participates in them. Level 3 interventions provide healthy lifestyle interventions, promoting physical activity, maintaining a healthy weight, and providing dietetics, mental health, or smoking cessation support.

Interventions are directed at the individual, with behavioral change as the primary focus. Digital apps offering health coaching are increasingly providing direct intervention support, placing individuals in a healthy digital environment aware of the importance of a healthy lifestyle, and increasing the ability and likelihood of patients to follow care plans. In reality, affordability and accessibility are critical components of healthy environments that provide the most significant inertia to change.

Level 4

Specific, system-targeted interventions focus on dysfunctional physiological systems. Examples include bariatric surgery for patients diagnosed with morbid obesity or pharmacological interventions for hypertension. Most patients in a level 4 intervention are in stage C or D of health. Ultimately, methods of evaluating the success of precision healthcare could well include the number of people the approach can support from entering stages C and D of health in the first place.

Level 4 interventions delivered to individuals in stages A and B of health focus on optimizing behaviors, collection and feedback of data, and prevention of disease states, promoting a consumer approach to health and wellness that will evolve and improve the ability to deliver precision health.

Regardless of the stage of health or level of intervention required when an individual enters the P5H continuum model, the objective is to prevent future disease risks and adverse events, treat underlying causes, and improve lifestyle behaviors. As such, all intervention levels can and should be delivered at all stages of health.

Summary

Healthcare is shifting from a reactive model to a proactive model to address the growing burden of chronic disease and health in its totality and the societal impact of illness. Attempts to make healthcare more predictive, preventive, personalized, participatory, and scalable to a population level are significantly improving health and well-being across the health continuum.

Precision lifestyle medicine is fundamental to the success of efforts to prevent and control costly chronic conditions, improve the health of populations, and eliminate health disparities. At the same time, system-level precision health approaches are transforming the way we understand common morbidities, why and how they are related, and, similarly, how we can reverse some, if not all, conditions, whether through genetics, environment, or behaviors. The P5H continuum provides such a framework, classifying four distinct levels of health and intervention. Not only does this approach encourage the maintenance of homeostasis, but it also promotes wellness and longevity, the foci of precision health.

CHAPTER 3

Data and the Digital Phenotype

For treatments to improve an individual's state of wellness at all points in the healthcare continuum, they must center around available data to provide patients with as-precise care as possible. The more that datasets are generated, linked, and utilized, the higher the accuracy of precision care. Data collection extends beyond genetics to various unconnected, fragmented sources that may not typically be considered related to health and disease.

Data is the fundamental requirement to realizing the ambition of precision health, and understandably, patients and healthcare professionals alike are excited by the prospect. A study conducted with a group of more than 4,000 patients with long-term conditions in 2022 found that one in three patients are happy to share their data with their healthcare professionals.[1] In its current guise, precision health is driven by the enormous potential of big data and artificial intelligence. Collecting large quantities of data with clinical confirmation of health status and diagnoses enables sophisticated algorithms, increasing the chances of correct diagnoses and potentially lowering costs that underline key outputs of precision health.

---

[1] Summers, C., Griffiths, F., Cave, J. and Panesar, A., 2022. Understanding the Security and Privacy Concerns About the Use of Identifiable Health Data in the Context of the COVID-19 Pandemic: Survey Study of Public Attitudes Toward COVID-19 and Data-Sharing. JMIR Formative Research, 6(7), p.e29337.

© Arjun Panesar 2023
A. Panesar, *Precision Health and Artificial Intelligence*,
https://doi.org/10.1007/978-1-4842-9162-7_3

Data Forms and Types

To fully understand the nature of data, we must first grasp its nature. Data can be characterized by form and type.

Forms

Data can take many forms such as characters, text, words, numbers, images, sound, and video, and it falls into two classifications: structured and unstructured. Structured data typically refers to something stored in a database or spreadsheet in a structure that follows a model or schema.

Readings from embedded sensors, smartphones, smartwatches, and IoT devices are forms of structured data—whether that be the provision of blood glucose readings, steps walked, calories burned, heart rate, or blood pressure. Unstructured data refers to everything else. Notes on medical records, communications, and social media are a few examples of unstructured data that hold considerable prospects. The lack of a predefined model or schema structure makes data compilation and interpretation a resource-intensive task concerning time and energy.

Nevertheless, the incorporation of unstructured data into the personalization of the healthcare experience provides a treasure trove of possibilities. More than 656,640,000 tweets are shared on Twitter, 734,400,000 comments are posted on Facebook, and 100 billion messages are sent on WhatsApp every 24 hours.[2] While it is known that our social networks can facilitate positive health outcomes by influencing our health behaviors, our interactions and communications are an area of data mining yet to be fully realized.

---

[2] Stout, D. (2022). Social Media Statistics: Top Social Networks by Popularity. [online] Dustin Stout. Available at: https://dustinstout.com/social-media-statistics/.

Types

There are several types of data. Big data is synonymous with AI and healthcare, referring to a collection of voluminous, traditional, and digital data sources for discovery and analysis. Big data has three core key characteristics: volume, variety and velocity. In other words, there's a lot of it. Through big data analytics, one can uncover hidden patterns, unknown correlations, trends, preferences, and additional information to help make better and more informed decisions. Figure 3-1 shows the three Vs of big data.

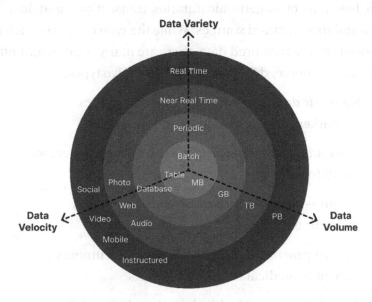

Figure 3-1. *The three Vs of data*

Machine learning and AI provide many techniques that data scientists can apply to datasets for this very purpose. Conversely, small data refers to N-equals-1 units of data that are accessible, informative, and actionable. Small data could include how many times a patient has been admitted into emergency care or whether they attended a scheduled appointment.

While data may be small in size, it does not lack value. The last few years have seen a shift toward including small data analytics to improve clinical and administrative processes and identify cost savings. Precision health seeks to deliver N-equals-1 care at scale.

Sources of Data

The data-driven understanding required to deliver individualized care is obtained from various data sets, including clinical repositories, electronic health records, genomic libraries, transactions, and data from structured and unstructured sources. While the type of data will fall into heterogeneous or unstructured data, there are many sources for both. Regardless of the source, data typically is one of five types.

- *Biometric data*: Fingerprints, genetics, -omics, biomarkers driven from apps and wearables

- *Web and social media data*: Clicks, history, behaviors, health forums

- *Machine-to-machine data*: Sensors, wearables, environment

- *Human-generated data*: Email, paper documents, electronic medical records, behaviors

- *Transaction data*: Health claim data, billing data

Precision health leverages data from various sources to understand the state of a human. Beyond -omics data, the ubiquitous use of the Internet and the widespread availability of smartphones adds rich clinical and biological data that can significantly enhance the understanding of an individual. Clinical data is supported with behavioral and social data. Lifestyle, environment, medical records, and medical insurance data can all be used to enable precision health. Given that a person with type 2 diabetes spends 3 hours with their clinician and the rest of their time is spent self-managing their condition, the potential opportunities enabled by more comprehensive data sources are self-evident.[3] For instance, there is no nonethical reason Google Maps could not give walking directions based on avoiding obesogenic-promoting restaurants or advertising to people who require weight management support or exhibit eating disorders. The question regarding incorporating new data sources is of morality rather than relevance.

As innovation in wearable devices and sensors continues, so does their implementation and application within clinical healthcare. Table 3-1 explores some common data types and sources. The key to maximizing clinical value from wearables within precision health is their integration into the broader data ecosystem and the rationale for data inclusion.

Table 3-1. *Common Data Types and Sources*

Data Type	Source	Example	Characteristics
Biometric	Genetic test Biomarker test	Genetic at-home testing (23andme)	Structured data. Owned by the patient.
Web and social media	Patient health, behaviors and sentiment	Social media Smartphones Web forums Communities, patient registries Health apps	Most data is unstructured or semistructured.

(continued)

---

[3] Milne, N. and Di Rosa, F., 2020. The diabetes review: A guide to the basics. Updated December 2020. Journal of Diabetes Nursing, 24(6).

Table 3-1. (*continued*)

Data Type	Source	Example	Characteristics
Machine-to-machine data	Patient health data	Sensors Blood glucose meters Smartphones Fitness trackers ImagesHealth apps	Structured data reported by devices. Software typically utilizes standard protocols. Sensor data is high velocity.
Human-generated data	Clinical data Pharmaceutical and R&D data	Electronic health recordPatient registries Clinical data Blood testsImages (scans, etc.)	Structured in nature. Owned by providers
Transactional data	Events and transactions logs	Health information exchanges Claims data Expenses data	Structured in nature. May require preprocessing to become useful data

Sensors

Intelligent sensing technologies can provide tremendous value to clinical services and insights into an individual's state of health. Sensors fall into two categories: worn or wearables and nonwearable sensors.

More than 40 percent of U.S. consumers now own a wearable device.[4] Wearable technologies are becoming more common, affordable, and sophisticated, moving past fashion accessories and activity tracking. Wearable sensors provide greater accuracy in geolocation and health signals; however, they are typically more intrusive than nonwearable sensors, which

---

[4] Statista. (n.d.). Wearable device ownership 2021. [online] Available at: `https://www.statista.com/forecasts/1101101/wearable-devices-ownership-in-selected-countries`.

are less invasive and can monitor activities across environments such as home, work, recreation areas, and transport with no interference to an individual's daily routines.

As sensors become smaller, embeddable, biodegradable, and constantly connected, they play increasingly critical roles in patient care. Their structured data is apt for research, machine learning, and analytics, as shown in Figure 3-2.

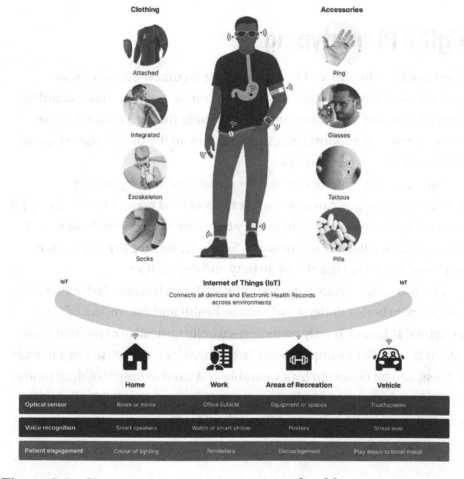

Figure 3-2. *Smart sensor usage in precision health*

The ubiquity of 5G communications is enabling smart care to evolve. Sensors within the home, workplace, transport, and urban areas can capture and transmit data, including behaviors, location, interactions, and communications. While this also conjures images of an Orwellian future, the power of using moment-by-moment health and behavioral data to optimize a person's state of wellness is not only revolutionary; it's gradually becoming a reality.

Digital Phenotyping

When available health and behavioral data is combined with social platforms and other interactions, a more comprehensive understanding of behavioral and social domains is achievable through a data-intense environment that supports precision health and the digital phenotype of health and, conversely, disease.

Because taking photos of food for social media has grown in popularity, dietitians can now use pictures of food taken from health apps or social media to understand dietary habits more precisely than a food diary or standardized questionnaire. Similarly, social platform use has been used to predict the risk of anxiety and depression.

The use of data from nontraditional domains has enabled digital healthcare to better understand human health and the impact of behaviors, although is only sometimes wholly indicative of the real-time state of health. For example, heart rate variability (HRV), used as a marker of stress, can be collected by a wearable and used to optimize drug intake.

Digital phenotyping is the process of inferring an individual's behavior from the digital data generated through interactions with electronic hardware and software.[5, 6] When determined to be clinically relevant, the power of data can provide insights into an individual's lifestyle, socio-demographics, psychology, and environment. This form of digital phenotyping has proven successful in psychiatry and type 2 diabetes. Figure 3-3 provides a diagrammatic representation of deep digital phenotyping.

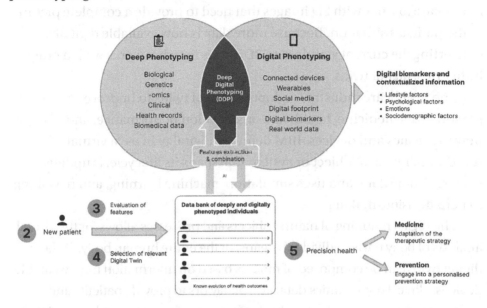

Figure 3-3. *Deep digital phenotyping*

[5] Spinazze, P., Rykov, Y., Bottle, A. and Car, J., 2019. Digital phenotyping for assessment and prediction of mental health outcomes: a scoping review protocol. BMJ open, 9(12), p.e032255.
[6] Fagherazzi, G., 2020. Deep digital phenotyping and digital twins for precision health: time to dig deeper. Journal of Medical Internet Research, 22(3), p.e16770.

Digital Twin

Many industries have used simulation and 3D modeling for developing and testing new products. Physical crash tests, for example, are rarely performed in the automotive industry, as these are now primarily performed in a virtual environment. However, it is still common practice in healthcare to work with 2D images that need to provide a complete picture of the patient's situation. Because more data is now available digitally, converting the current standard to 3D allows for what works well in other industries: digital twins.

The healthcare industry is adopting digital twins to improve personalized medicine, healthcare organization performance, and new medicines and devices. IBM defines a digital twin as "a virtual representation of an object or system that spans its lifecycle, is updated from real-time data, and uses simulation, machine learning, and reasoning to help decision-making."[7]

The digital mapping of natural objects and processes allows for the virtual analysis of body parts, individual organs, or the entire human body. Today's digital twins can be composed of models based on information from wearable devices, clinical data, -omics data, and behaviors to provide patients and clinicians with empowering feedback. Furthermore, results can be simulated under the same conditions as the tangible counterpart by training the models with actual patient data. While digital twins are still a relatively new concept within healthcare, the field of digital twins is expanding rapidly with advances in data connectivity, AI, and AR/VR. Aware that a one-size-fits-all approach to healthcare is inefficient, there is growing support for scaling digital twins from isolated research projects to mass personalization, as is familiar with today's customer data and advertising platforms.

---

[7] IBM Business Operations Blog. (2020). Cheat sheet: What is Digital Twin? Internet of Things blog. [online] Available at: `https://www.ibm.com/blogs/internet-of-things/iot-cheat-sheet-digital-twin`.

A digital twin would be a virtual patient with similar or close characteristics to a new patient seen during a clinical visit, and for whom the health status, risks of complications, and disease progressions are known. In the not-too-distant future, each patient will have a digital twin, obtained thanks to deep digital phenotyping, represented by the average characteristics of its closest cluster group. We are moving away from representing diabetes patients by their HbA1c and fasting blood glucose levels to real-time data analytics enabling differentiation between subclinical types of diabetes. It is not long before we have the deep digital phenotype of individuals with millions of data points comprised of clinical, biological, genetic, sociological, psychological, communications, and real-world data, revolutionizing how we understand health and disease.

Computer science, behavioral psychology, bioinformatics, and epidemiology are core themes. From multi-omics approaches to unsupervised deep learning algorithms, along with the proper computational power, we now have the appropriate tools to deal with the diversity and quantity of information and move from coarsely stratified groups to refined, small groups of individuals defined by numerous features.

Data Challenges

There is a growing number of reliable, practical, and actionable measures of health behavior, mental health, patient preferences, and social determinants of health available today that could expand the range of valuable data to construct more fully informed personalized health treatments.

Patients and providers can make more co-informed, individualized decisions about healthcare options by collecting and rapidly summarizing critical results based on these factors. For this to occur, several key inertias still need to be overcome.

Measurement and Completeness

It is essential to consider the completeness of available data, inaccuracies, and imprecisions in self-reported data that can significantly skew results at both the individual and population levels. Missing data is a potential entrance for bias within a system.

Additionally, until very recently, patient-reported measures have been regarded as unscientific or impractical to use in real-world healthcare. Nonetheless, recent research has shown that clinicians can efficiently collect patient-reported health behavior, mental health, and preference data with little deviation from clinically collected data.[8]

Lack of Data on Social Determinants of Health

The social determinants of health have a huge impact on whether a patient will engage within healthcare. Research has demonstrated that the social determinants of health have approximately twice the impact on healthcare access and outcomes than medical intervention.[9, 10] As access to healthcare data at scale becomes viable, ensuring that data on social and environmental determinants of health such as ethnicity,

---

[8] Løvaas, K.F., Cooper, J.G., Sandberg, S., Røraas, T. and Thue, G., 2015. Feasibility of using self-reported patient data in a national diabetes register. BMC Health Services Research, 15(1), pp.1–7.

[9] Hill, J., Nielsen, M. and Fox, M.H., 2013. Understanding the social factors that contribute to diabetes: a means to informing health care and social policies for the chronically ill. The Permanente Journal, 17(2), p.67.

[10] Braveman, P. and Gottlieb, L., 2014. The social determinants of health: it's time to consider the causes of the causes. Public health reports, 129(1_suppl2), pp.19–31.

gender, education, co-morbidities, income, employment, literacy, and neighborhood is linked to biomedical data will contribute significant improvements in healthcare for people and populations.

Examples of technologies that address social determinants include behavioral change platforms and wellness programs that cater to ethnicity, gender, race, religion, and language. While positive signs are emerging in addressing social determinants of health, the challenge remains the scarcity of available data.

Privacy and Security

The collection and use of health and nonstandard data, such as point-in-time ecological assessments via social media or GPS monitoring, raise serious privacy, security, and ethical concerns. Many healthcare services have rapidly digitalized during COVID to maintain continuity of care. Data collection and dissemination provided critical support for defending against the spread of the novel virus since the beginning of the pandemic. However, more needs to be known about public perceptions of and attitudes toward data use, privacy, and security.

A recent study in 2022, which sought to understand better people's willingness to share data, received 4,764 responses showing the public attention on the topic.[11] More people are more comfortable sharing anonymized data than personally identifiable data. People reported feeling comfortable sharing data that we're able to benefit others; 66 percent would share personally identifiable data if its purpose were deemed beneficial for the health of others, and 63.9 percent would consent to

---

[11] Summers, C., Griffiths, F., Cave, J. and Panesar, A., 2022. Understanding the Security and Privacy Concerns About the Use of Identifiable Health Data in the Context of the COVID-19 Pandemic: Survey Study of Public Attitudes Toward COVID-19 and Data-Sharing. JMIR Formative Research, 6(7), p.e29337

share personal, sensitive health data with government or health authority organizations. Nevertheless, there were serious concerns over data use.

More than a quarter of respondents stated that they did not trust any organization to protect their data, and 54 percent reported concerns about the implications of sharing personal information. Alarmingly, just under two-thirds of respondents noted concerns about the provisions of appropriate legislation that seeks to prevent data misuse and hold organizations accountable in the case of data misuse. Data owners (people using services) are increasingly crucial to ethical and regulatory aspects regarding data security, privacy, and trust.

It is challenging to safely aggregate and anonymize data while preserving all of the multidimensional statistical properties and relationships that exist within it. Regardless, privacy must precede the sharing and exchange of data between organizations. Privacy could take the form, for instance, of synthetic or anonymized data that researchers can share freely and algorithms that protect individual-level identification. Academia, organizations, governments, and regulators have more to do to engage the public with ethical and transparent data sharing.

Transparent research, including informed consent, co-developed patient and clinician solutions, and engagement between stakeholders at each step of the product lifecycle, is required to build trust as digital phenotyping goes past traditional data sources and consumes a variety of big data for large and varied populations. The nascency of legal guidance in this area suggests a need for humanitarian guidelines for data responsibility during disaster relief operations such as pandemics and for involving the public in their development.

Cost

Precision entails an emphasis on data that is not conventionally tied to health and illness, as well as a focus on genetics. However, regardless of the health system, resource cost must be considered as a significant variable in precision medicine. Health monitoring can quickly become costly, so cost-effective strategies must be identified and implemented throughout the care continuum.

For instance, while there are static biomarkers (e.g., a specific genetic variant), others change over time and need to be evaluated periodically. Ideally, many markers can predict future health status with high precision; researchers should identify a cost-effective set to guarantee the same performance with minimal burden. It is reasonable to suggest that there will, at some point in the future, exist sufficient data to provide an almost complete picture of precision health for an individual without requiring anything more than genetic and lifestyle data. The challenge will be to achieve that without exorbitant cost.

Disconnected from Data

While people may have access to their wearable and device data through services such as Apple Health or Google Fit, they still need to be in control of their medical data. Electronic health record systems and data repositories stand isolated and do not exploit the benefits of connected care.

Limited Adoption of Common Data Models

Data harmonization is a massive digital challenge, and future standards must continue to promote shared understanding for precision care to be realized. There is a requirement for unified structural and semantic representations and data models to encourage interoperability and connectivity between health ecosystems. However, no such model exists entirely, with a broad range of data models and terminology used within nations, vendors, and internationally, with some organizations without data standards.

OpenEHR is an excellent example of a standard data model in the nascency of being adopted across large-scale healthcare services. The platform provides a product and vendor-neutral structured method for defining health data, data content, and terminology that enables care participation, coordination, and collaboration.

Expanding Beyond Qualitative Data

Most developments within precision health have been focused on -omics and device-driven historical data that is used to train predictive algorithms. Precision health has become synonymous with quantitative research, with very little focus on qualitative health data yet to be utilized in precision health research. Excluding qualitative data, mainly unstructured data may need to include the most precise and informative data on human behaviors, opinions, and details of people, among other contextual factors.

A Paradigm for Acting on Data

Collecting data is for taking action. This can be modeled using the Sense, Think, Act paradigm. Whether a human, artificially intelligent agent, or hybrid conducts the thinking, what differentiates data value creation is how these aspects are used to deliver meaningful value that engages their ecosystem, optimizes operations, and creates new efficiencies and opportunities. Figure 3-4 provides an approach for digital transformation known as Sense, Think, Act.

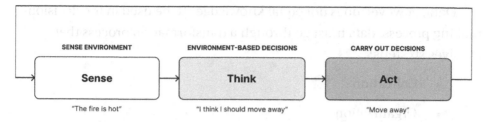

Figure 3-4. *The Sense, Think, Act paradigm of digital transformation*

Sense refers to the continuous collection of data from multiple sources in real time. Think refers to the aggregation, analysis, and development of information and knowledge from data. Act refers to an action that takes place with an awareness of the contextual landscape from data sources available to the agent conducting an activity. It is from these actions that measures are taken to transform the information into value.

Turning Data into Information, Knowledge, and Wisdom

IBM reports that more than 1 TB of data is created daily, but less than 1 percent of the data is being used.[12] Data's value is demonstrated in the ability to convert it into information that can drive actionable insight to drive behaviors and workflows. Data analytics is a theme within data science that seeks to draw information from raw data sources. Real-time analytics supports agile insight discovery and analysis at the point of decision.

---

[12] manufacturingdigital.com. (2020). IBM: the potential of smart manufacturing. [online] Available at: https://manufacturingdigital.com/technology/ibm-potential-smart-manufacturing.

Data, however, does not equal knowledge. To be used in the decision-making process, data must go through a transformation process that involves six steps:

- Collection

- Organization

- Processing

- Integration

- Reporting

- Utilization

Data is transformed into information that enables knowledge if interpreted correctly. The Data, Information, Knowledge, Wisdom (DIKW) pyramid is a common model for thinking about data transformation and value creation. Figure 3-5 is an adaptation of the DIKW model, which shows how data is relevant to digital transformation.

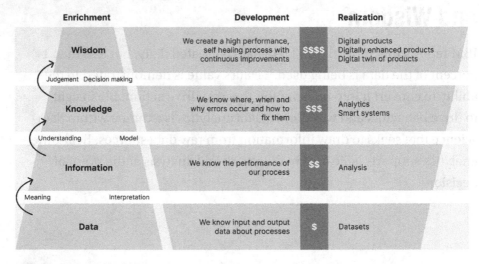

Figure 3-5. *Using data to enable information, knowledge, and wisdom*

Data enrichment is transforming data into information, knowledge, and wisdom. Value development refers to how an opportunity's value is developed by applying those transformations. Value realization refers to value development regarding outputs, products, services, and outcomes.

As the scale and importance of data increases, he time between data creation to insight and action needs to be reduced. There is substantial economic value in reducing the time from a detected event to an automatic response, which can identify fraudulent transactions, improve service capacity by freeing up hospital beds when patients are immediately ready for discharge, and spot signs of deteriorating health before a catastrophe.

Summary

To fully realize the potential inherent in the big data we can now generate, we must change the way we work. Creating collaborative networks and sharing data and models are more important than ever, and this process increasingly necessitates bridging to less traditional collaborating specialties such as engineering, computer science, and industry.

While data collection and analysis can provide substantial insight, digital phenotyping is a powerful tool for assessing individual health conditions and studying wider public health trends.

As stakeholders act on the insights and knowledge generated through digital systems, they will produce better engagement with patients and clinicians, better products and services, and new applications of precision health. Making the most of big data will be a challenge, but the potential rewards are even more remarkable. In the next chapter, we will explore the foundations of artificial intelligence and its application to precision health.

CHAPTER 4

Artificial Intelligence and Machine Learning in Precision Health

Artificial intelligence refers to any cognitive ability exhibited by a nonhuman agent. The five fundamental components of artificial intelligence are learning, reasoning, problem-solving, perception, and language comprehension. AI has already surpassed human ability when it comes to performing tasks such as learning, vision, and logical reasoning.[1] Machine learning is a subset of AI where computer models are trained to learn from their actions and environment over time to improve. Algorithms adapt to the presentation of new data and discovery and, through machine learning, get iteratively better at tasks without having to be explicitly programmed to do so. Machine learning is AI that can adapt autonomously with minimum human intervention.

Deep learning is a subset of machine learning that uses artificial neural networks to simulate the human brain's learning process. The process is called *deep learning* due to additional layers that are added to a deep learning function when learning from data. Layers within the function are

---

[1] Garnelo, M. and Shanahan, M., 2019. Reconciling deep learning with symbolic artificial intelligence: representing objects and relations. Current Opinion in Behavioral Sciences, 29, pp.17–23.

© Arjun Panesar 2023
A. Panesar, *Precision Health and Artificial Intelligence*,
https://doi.org/10.1007/978-1-4842-9162-7_4

called *neurons*. When a deep learning model learns, it simply modifies weights, or neurons, using an optimization function. Figure 4-1 shows a component analysis on AI.

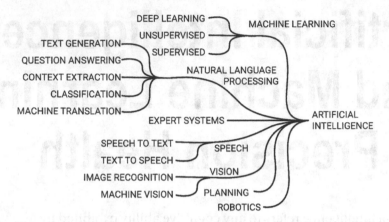

Figure 4-1. *Components of AI*

Natural language processing (NLP) is the capacity of systems to analyze, comprehend, and produce human language, including speech and text. Natural language interpretation is difficult because human language is innately ambiguous—language, pronunciation, expression, and perception. To analyze and understand natural language, the grammatical structure of sentences and the meaning of words are broken down into bits so that they may be studied and comprehended in context. NLP blends AI with computational linguistics and computer science.

Integrating AI approaches such as machine learning, deep learning, and techniques such as NLP to tackle the challenges of scalability and high dimensionality of data into actionable knowledge is becoming the foundation of precision medicine. The ubiquity of sensor-based technologies such as smartphones and wearable devices enables a new age of health AI where real-time decisions are made based on vital signs, environment, and behaviors. However, the benefits of AI still require addressing against the technical, legal, and ethical challenges that remain to ensure that stakeholders can realize the precision health ecosystem.

The hypothesis-generating approach to science is best viewed as a complementary means of identifying and inferring meaning from data patterns rather than simply extending what has always been done. A growing number of AI methods allow these patterns or trends to be learned directly from the data rather than being prespecified by researchers based on prior knowledge.

The Three Types of AI

Any AI application falls into one of three types of intelligence based on how well they can replicate human characteristics, the technology to achieve this, application, and theory of mind.

Artificial Narrow Intelligence

To date, the only artificial intelligence humans have successfully realized is artificial narrow intelligence (ANI), also known as weak or narrow AI. Narrow AI excels at performing a single task. Think of speech recognition, spam filters, autonomous cars, movie recommendations, and software to support facial recognition. Large volumes of data can be processed in seconds using narrow AI algorithms without accumulating fatigue.

There are two types of narrow AI: reactive and memory-limited. Reactive AI has no storage capabilities, simulating the human mind's ability to respond to stimuli without prior experience. In contrast, most AI solutions use limited-memory AI, which has data storage and learning capabilities that allow machines to use preliminary data to inform future decisions. Deep learning, for example, tailors future experiences based on previously stored data.

Artificial General Intelligence

Artificial general intelligence (AGI) or strong AI is the concept of a human-like agent with general intelligence that can learn and apply its knowledge and experience to solve problems. This form of AI acts, thinks, and understands in a manner indistinguishable from human behavior. Strong AI revolves around the theory of mind AI framework, which details the ability to discern other intelligent entities' needs, emotions, beliefs, and thought processes. Theory of mind AI is not about replication or simulation; instead, it is about teaching machines to understand humans truly. There are currently no notable examples of strong AI.

Artificial Superintelligence

A theoretical concept currently, artificial superintelligence (ASI) goes beyond mimicking human intelligence and behavior. It is when agents are aware of themselves and exceed the capacity of human ability and intelligence. Whether this is inevitable is generally a question of ethics and morality rather than technology.

A Brief Introduction to Machine Learning

Machine learning exemplifies data mining principles but can also infer correlations and learn from them to apply to new algorithms.

Regardless of the type of AI, the goal is to mimic the ability to learn like a human through experience and achieve the assigned task without or with minimal external assistance. Machine learning tasks can be *supervised*, where models are developed upon example inputs; *unsupervised*, where models determine their structure from an input; and *partially supervised*, a combination of the two.

Framework for Machine Learning

Regardless of the approach taken, once a problem has been framed, a typical AI or machine learning workflow would generally comprise the following:

- *Data preparation*: Involving data exploration, analysis, insight, and cleaning

- *Training*: Choosing learning method(s), applying them to create a model, and attempting to optimize the models created

- *Testing*: An objective assessment of the method and results

- *Dissemination*: Reporting the results of an evaluation to stakeholders and ensuring explainability

- *Deployment*: Releasing the trained machine learning model, monitoring ongoing usage and accuracy

The training phase involves maximizing the performance of an algorithm through adjustments to key parameters (or tuning) that alter the algorithm's behavior. A parameter is a variable utilized by the model where the model can estimate the value from the dataset. The volume and type of parameters are crucial aspects of any algorithm. While there is no data like more data, it's ultimately of no use if the data is trash—additionally, both the time and resources required to train a model increase with parameter dimensionality. If training on a small set of parameters, models risk missing subtle trends and patterns, while large volumes of data can cause algorithms difficulty identifying valuable patterns.

The testing phase then assesses the tuning of parameters through their performance to ensure the model is generalizable, which is the goal of all algorithms. Mathematically, one can understand this as attempting to minimize a cost function on training and test data so that models perform confidently and can be deployed in the real world.

Table 4-1 lists some examples of learning approaches and algorithms.

Table 4-1. *Examples of Learning Approaches and Algorithms*

Supervised	Unsupervised	NLP
• Support vector machines • Naïve Bayes • Gaussian Bayes • K-nearest neighbors (KNN) • Logistic regression	• Apriori algorithm • FP-growth (also known as frequent pattern growth) • Hidden Markov model • Principal component analysis (PCA) • Singular value decomposition (SVD) • K-means • Neural networks • Deep learning	• C4.5 • K-means • Support vector machines • Apriori • EM (expectation–maximization) • PageRank • AdaBoost • kNN • Naïve Bayes • Classification and regression trees (CART)

High generalization leads to overfitting or underfitting. If a model performs better on training datasets than on unseen test sets, then the model is likely to be overfitting. Cross-validation is a technique to employ to measure against overfitting. Further still, training with more data may help algorithms infer hypotheses better.

Underfitting is simple to detect, as it will have poor performance. Bias represents the error the model has from learning from erroneous data. Bias measures how far off, in general, these models' predictions are from the actual correct value or true signal. Increasing model complexity to determine subtle signals reduces bias but introduces variance, which determines the variability of model predictions around a data point. Ensuring model generalizability is a trade-off between bias and variance (Figure 4-2). Wherever possible, it is better to keep it simple than over-engineer and build complex and expensive machine learning models that are difficult to explain and disseminate.

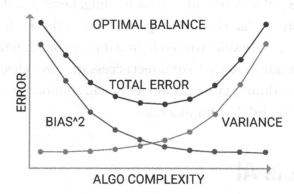

Figure 4-2. *Finding optimal algorithmic balance*

Software and Toolkits

It is easier than ever to tap into the power of machine learning with easy-to-implement libraries and frameworks. Healthcare providers are moving slowly toward sophisticated toolkits to utilize the massive real-time data stream created by patients, driven by established healthcare providers, startups, and enterprises, and academia. Open-source toolkits support machine learning by providing accessible and ready-to-use code for common algorithms. Most are available for Python, the programming language favored for developing machine learning algorithms.

Scikit-learn is a Python module containing image processing and machine learning techniques built on SciPy and enables algorithms for clustering, classification, and regression, such as naïve Bayes, decision trees, random forests, k-means, and support vector machines. NLTK, or Natural Language Toolkit, is a collection of libraries used in natural language processing. The NLTK enables the foundations for expert systems such as tokenization, stemming, tagging, parsing, and classification. Genism is a library for use on unstructured text, Scrapy provides open-source data mining, and TensorFlow is a popular Alphabet-backed open-source library of data computations optimized for deep learning. It enables multilayered neural networks and quick training. Keras and PyTorch are libraries for building deep learning algorithms with TensorFlow.

WEKA is a software suite written in Java that enables interaction via a graphical user interface (GUI) or direct access that provides, similar to sci-kit-learn, algorithms, visualization tools, and support for a range of machine learning and data mining tasks.

Explainable AI

Initiatives such as the General Data Protection Regulation (GDPR) in the European Union, the Health Insurance Portability and Accountability Act (HIPAA) in the United States, and the Privacy Act in Australia have pushed the conversation about explainable AI in healthcare into the mainstream. While AI systems have been shown to outperform humans in various tasks, lack of explainability continues to spark criticism. Explainability involves understanding how a particular AI-driven decision is made. AI algorithms are sophisticated mathematical models for which the explainability of complex optimization processes becomes nontrivial. The benefits of improving trust and transparency in AI do not just benefit end users but also support the overall accuracy and generalizability of growing systems.

Applications of AI Assisted Precision Health in Practice

AI-driven precision healthcare technologies promise to improve the quality of care and outcomes across the board. As large amounts of diverse data from health studies and research are generated, it will become increasingly more challenging to differentiate between precision medicine and public health. While we may be years away from realizing the full potential of precision healthcare, early efforts are addressing significant challenges and demonstrating the critical role that AI technology and computational power advances can play across various themes.

Clinical Decision Support

Clinical decision support tools have been used for years. Still, many of them have needed to be more stand-alone solutions and adequately integrated into the clinical point-of-care devices used by providers. AI-led clinical decision support systems can improve the diagnosis, treatment, and prognosis of a particular medical condition, by predicting the probability of a medical outcome or the risk for a specific disease based on biomedical imaging data. Numerous studies have shown that AI and other analytics tools can accurately predict kidney disease, identify breast cancer, and forecast leukemia remission rates.[2] AI systems have outperformed state-of-the-art methods and received FDA approval for various clinical diagnostics, particularly imaging-based diagnostics.[3] The availability

---

[2] Huang, S., Yang, J., Fong, S. and Zhao, Q., 2020. Artificial intelligence in cancer diagnosis and prognosis: Opportunities and challenges. Cancer letters, 471, pp.61–71.

[3] Karandikar, P., Massaad, E., Hadzipasic, M., Kiapour, A., Joshi, R.S., Shankar, G.M. and Shin, J.H., 2022. Machine learning applications of surgical imaging for the diagnosis and treatment of spine disorders: Current state of the art. Neurosurgery, 90(4), pp.372–382.

of large datasets for training, such as extensive collections of annotated medical images or large functional genomics datasets, is driving this surge in productivity, along with advances in AI algorithms and the GPU systems used to train them.

With the correct data, integration methods, and team, machine learning has the potential to improve the usefulness of clinical decision-support tools and help providers deliver optimal care. The biggest challenge in developing algorithms is gaining access to large amounts of data required to train models to suggest next steps for treatment, flag potential risks, and enhance service efficiency and capacity.

Behavioral Change Interventions and Lifestyle Medicine

Digital therapeutics refers to evidence-based therapeutic interventions for patients to prevent, manage, or treat a medical condition or disease. Digital therapeutics are typically considered mobile apps, but a growing number are available across platforms.[4] Digital therapeutics are distinguished from more general health and fitness apps by their clinical classification, intended audience specificity, demonstrated research, and impact. Patient-facing digital health applications (apps) provide the opportunity to change how individuals take responsibility for their health by enabling more effective delivery of health information, allowing better monitoring of health markers, and encouraging lifestyle behavior change. Several systematic reviews suggest that app-based interventions can improve diet,

---

[4] Hatami, H., Deravi, N., Danaei, B., Zangiabadian, M., Shahidi Bonjar, A.H., Kheradmand, A. and Nasiri, M.J., 2022. Tele-medicine and improvement of mental health problems in COVID-19 pandemic: A systematic review. International Journal of Methods in Psychiatric Research, 31(3), p.e1924.

physical activity, and sedentary behavior.[5] Controlled trials still need to be conducted to confirm whether multicomponent interventions are more effective than stand-alone apps.

With most disease risk coming from modifiable risk factors, precision behavioral change and lifestyle interventions delivered through digital therapeutics hold enormous potential to contribute to public health prevention efforts to successfully and efficiently promote population health, control healthcare costs, and eliminate health inequalities. For most people, the key to improved health isn't a diet or exercise program based on specious conclusions from sequencing your genome, analyzing your microbiome, or surveilling your smartphone. Instead, it's figuring out how to remain motivated when adopting and maintaining positive health behaviors.

Precision behavioral change and lifestyle interventions in the form of therapeutic intervention, behavioral change coaching, and biomedical data feedback and sensors enable wellness to be truly patient-centered, solution-focused, and precise. Importantly, precision behavior change interventions have been shown to work.[6, 7] Numerous studies show precision health platforms engage people across cultures, provide equivalent care to face-to-face care, and improve quality of life and weight loss.[8]

---

[5] Hutchesson, M.J., Gough, C., Müller, A.M., Short, C.E., Whatnall, M.C., Ahmed, M., Pearson, N., Yin, Z., Ashton, L.M., Maher, C. and Staiano, A.E., 2021. eHealth interventions targeting nutrition, physical activity, sedentary behavior, or obesity in adults: A scoping review of systematic reviews. Obesity Reviews.

[6] Summers, C., Tobin, S. and Unwin, D., 2021. Evaluation of the Low Carb Program Digital Intervention for the Self-Management of Type 2 Diabetes and Prediabetes in an NHS England General Practice: Single-Arm Prospective Study. JMIR diabetes, 6(3), p.e25751.

[7] Hanson, P., Summers, C., Panesar, A., Oduro-Donkor, D., Lange, M., Menon, V., & Barber, T. M. (2021). Low Carb Program Health App Within a Hospital-Based Obesity Setting: Observational Service Evaluation. JMIR Formative Research, 5(9), e29110.

[8] Scott, E., Shehata, M., Panesar, A., Summers, C., & Dale, J. (2022). The Low Carb Program for people with type 2 diabetes and pre-diabetes: a mixed methods feasibility study of signposting from general practice. BJGP open, 6(1).

Behavioral change platforms can support learning and adopting healthy habits in the real world and the virtual world at all times, using traditional in-platform and immersive virtual and augmented experiences to reinforce learning and maintain behavioral changes.[9] People are consistently guided to lead healthy lives in a tailored manner that maximizes the chances of reaching health goals or target measurements. Most precision health behavior change interventions depend on human-led, low-tech personalization and rely on data rules alone; most platforms still need to fully consider the interaction between people's behaviors and social and environmental contexts. As behavioral change interventions improve, they will increasingly go beyond personalization according to current behaviors and demographics and consider individuals' genetic profiles and social and environmental context in real time.

The highly variable response to obesity therapies justifies treatment strategies best suited to individual patients. A precision obesity solution would combine genetic testing, environment interactions, epigenetics, metabolomics, microbiome, pharmacogenomics, nutrigenetics, nutrigenomics, and deep digital phenotyping with a wrap-around behavioral change intervention to support adherence, health optimization, and remote monitoring.

From my own experiences, the most significant inertia in adopting behavior change interventions are stakeholders within the decision-making pathway who are critical of motivating people to engage with interventions and maintain them. Many healthcare providers have tried and often failed incentive programs for cigarette smoking, weight loss, and physical activity. Traditional healthcare systems are cynical and unaware of how to modify health behaviors. Digital engagement, however,

---

[9] Abdelhameed, F., Pearson, E., Hanson, P., Barber, T., Panesar, A. and Summers, C., 2022, May. Health outcomes following engagement with a digital health tool GroHealth app amongst people with type 2 diabetes. In Endocrine Abstracts (Vol. 81). Bioscientifica.

is distinct from engagement in health promotional activities. It is relatively straightforward to engage people digitally through an understanding of their basic measurements such as age, gender, and ethnicity. Through machine learning on large datasets, we can understand the behaviors and patterns exhibited by people exhibiting similar deep digital phenotypes to maximize the likelihood of engagement and long-term adherence from even the most unmotivated groups of people.

New Treatments, Definitions of Disease, and Points of Intervention

Vast networks of scientific and patient data will enable researchers to uncover new knowledge and essential disease insights, such as novel drug targets that can be expected to have a higher probability of success. These biomarkers can help characterize patients into subgroups likely to benefit from treatment and support the design of better clinical trials where suitable patients are recruited to participate and develop treatments for the real world. Large sets of -omics data and genomic biomarkers have the potential to uncover novel associations between molecular profiles and other clinical variables that would not have been identified otherwise, potentially leading to the identification of new clinically relevant subtypes in clinical trials. Figure 4-3 shows how precision health can be used to develop better treatments.

Current Healthcare
ONE TREATMENT FITS ALL

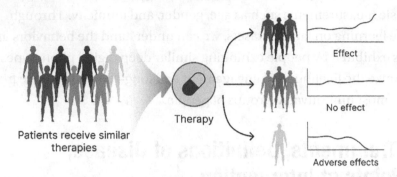

Patients receive similar
therapies

Therapy

Effect

No effect

Adverse effects

Future Healthcare
PERSONALIZED DIAGNOSTICS AND TREATMENT

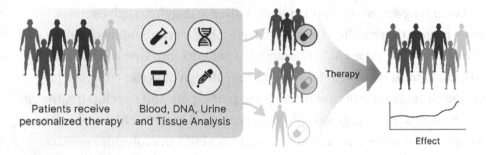

Patients receive
personalized therapy

Blood, DNA, Urine
and Tissue Analysis

Therapy

Effect

Figure 4-3. Precision treatments provide efficacious treatments for all patients

As data demonstrates previously unseen signals, new disease definitions are being defined. For example, behavioral change interventions have been shown to support weight loss, improve blood glucose control, and reverse cardiometabolic conditions such as type 2 diabetes and prediabetes.[10] Consequently, the definition of type 2 diabetes

---

[10] Saslow, L.R., Summers, C., Aikens, J.E. and Unwin, D.J., 2018. Outcomes of a digitally delivered low-carbohydrate type 2 diabetes self-management program: 1-year results of a single-arm longitudinal study. JMIR diabetes, 3(3), p.e9333.

has changed in many countries, supported by big data, from a chronic and progressive disease to a disease that patients can reverse.

Similarly, researchers can use machine-learning algorithms to predict potential future events such as depressive behavior and suicide risk. A model was trained by researchers at Vanderbilt University Medical Center using hospital admissions data, demographic data, and diagnostic history from just 5,000 patients to accurately predict whether an individual would risk taking their life in the proceeding seven days in 84 percent of cases and was able to accurately predict whether an individual would attempt suicide in the next two years in 80 percent of cases. When detected, patients can be escalated to emergency care and supported with intensive behavioral and mental health support.

Digital Twins

Digital twin instances and aggregates allow for the formulation and testing of novel hypotheses, in silico experiments and comparisons, and the discovery of new knowledge from the small data of one person to the big data of one or several populations by ensuring target populations are well represented in the corresponding digital twin representations.[11] Personalized heart models, for example, are used to aid clinical treatments for severe heart defects in newborns. Many virtual surgeries can be performed under the physician's supervision using digital twins to determine the best approach.

The characteristics of digital twins, such as digital thread tracing and tracking, enable highly personalized treatment pathways, better outcomes, and more explainable AI. Similar to the challenges AI and data analytics face, digital twins are affected by data availability and quality, data

---

[11] Kamel Boulos, M.N. and Zhang, P., 2021. Digital twins: from personalised medicine to precision public health. Journal of Personalized Medicine, 11(8), p.745.

integration and interoperability, data sharing, concerns about intellectual property, data privacy and security across platforms and systems, AI bias, explainability, and reproducibility.

AI reproducibility and bias reduction in intelligent digital twins can be achieved by ensuring that target populations are fairly represented in their respective digital twins and digital twin aggregates.

Health Promoting Chatbots

Research shows that AI chatbots demonstrate significant usability, feasibility, and acceptability worldwide.[12] With almost 100 percent uptime, chatbots are perfect for promoting and maintaining healthy behaviors, whether smoking cessation, better nutrition, or medication adherence. Health-promoting chatbots overcome digital telehealth limitations, such as unsustainability, low adherence, and inflexibility, by providing personalized on-demand support with higher levels of interactivity and sustainability.

Health-promoting chatbots collect data from various sources, including the user, analyze it using machine learning and natural language processing techniques, and provide the user with data outputs such as information, signposting behavioral change support, or escalation to more intensive support. Chatbots that promote health are already showing great promise in terms of saving time. Patients, for example, can communicate their symptoms via a messenger chat and receive live consultations without booking appointments or visiting facilities.

---

[12] Chen, J.S., Tran-Thien-Y, L. and Florence, D., 2021. Usability and responsiveness of artificial intelligence chatbot on online customer experience in e-retailing. International Journal of Retail & Distribution Management, 49(11), pp.1512–1531.

Voice Recognition

The human voice is a rich medium that serves as a primary communication source. Virtual/vocal assistants on smartphones or smart home devices such as connected speakers are now mainstream and have facilitated the numerous uses of voice-controlled search. For a good reason, too—speaking is one of the most natural, energy-efficient ways of interacting. As animals, we share insights about our emotions, fears, feelings, and excitation by modulating our voice's tone or pitch. Diseases can affect organs such as the heart, lungs, brain, muscles, or vocal folds, altering an individual's voice.

Voice-recognition algorithms process raw sound waves from human speech to recognize essential elements of speech; vocal biomarkers such as tempo, pitch, timbre, and volume; and more complex speech features such as spoken language, words, and sentences. The main applications of speech recognition thus far are voice command and virtual assistant systems.

Although voice-recognition algorithms are not yet widely used in clinical diagnostics, they have shown great promise in detecting neurological conditions that are often difficult to diagnose with traditional clinical tools. Because of its ability to reveal information about a person, such as their identity, demographics, ethnicity, or even their health status in cases of vocal biomarkers, voice data is considered sensitive.

Voice recognition has been used successfully to detect diseases that have a noticeable impact on speech, such as chronic pharyngitis, as well as diseases that have a less pronounced effect on speech, such as Alzheimer's disease, Parkinson's disease, major depressive disorder, posttraumatic stress disorder, and coronary artery disease. The same general speech-recognition strategies are used in these clinical applications. Still, the outcome targeted by the final classification step is a disease phenotype typically associated with speech characteristics (tone, tempo, pitch, and so on) rather than language content. The validation of vocal biomarkers against gold standards is mandatory for the safe use of voice to monitor health-related outcomes.

It is also vital to consider language and accent when using voice technologies or vocal biomarkers on a large scale. Otherwise, they could result in systemic biases toward people from certain regions, with different backgrounds, or with various accents and exacerbate the existing digital and socioeconomic divides. To limit bias toward under-represented groups of the population, voice technologies or vocal biomarkers must rely on algorithms trained on diverse datasets. Researchers must also improve the ability to process and understand natural language, relevance, and accuracy of voice assistant answers. Figure 4-4 gives examples of how vocal biomarkers can be used in health.

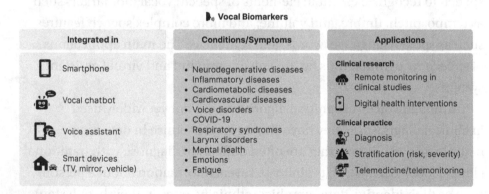

Figure 4-4. *Overview of the use of vocal biomarkers for health*

From audio to video, the field is moving. Adding images to voice data allows for better characterizing patients, emotions, and other health characteristics. The use of facial recognition and novel technologies, such as the smartphone camera combined with vocal biomarkers, makes remote health monitoring more precise and reliable. With the introduction of 5G networks and future updates, as well as an increasing number of smartphones and at-home devices with voice assistants, large vocal samples will be easier to collect and process.

As they say, a picture is worth a thousand words; and a video is worth a thousand pictures.

Summary

From the objective and thorough analysis of health data to identifying new long-term patterns and risk factors to aid diagnosis, machine learning, as a branch of AI, provides a myriad of opportunities to enhance medicine and healthcare. Further still, using AI in commercialized health systems offers a solution for patient-centered and personalized healthcare and well-being treatments. Nevertheless, machine learning applications to digital health have mainly been restricted to narrow domains. However, recent advancements in sensors and the Internet of Things mean we can now collect more data on users' broader physical and emotional states than ever.

As discussed in this chapter, there are many challenges to overcome, including significantly improving explainability and transparency, before we can expect more widespread adoption of AI in core healthcare services. Nonetheless, continued research in AI for digital health will help stimulate the overall drive of digital health and AI with substantial value for modern societies.

CHAPTER 5

Risks and Ethical Challenges of Precision Health

The goal of precision health necessitates extensive data collection on a patient's genetic characteristics, lifestyle, and environmental factors. While patients and professionals anticipate significant benefits from precision health and exhibit a positive attitude toward it, they also perceive risks from the convergence of next-generation sequencing, information technology, and AI. Many risks associated with AI have philosophical, moral, and ethical implications.

The clinical, technology, and academic communities have yet to solve the risks raised by traditional medical technologies. So, the rise of AI-driven precision health systems brings new and different dimensions to these challenges. Thankfully, several practices and themes are emerging that can help us navigate the complex world of morality unearthed by autonomous and intelligent systems.

© Arjun Panesar 2023
A. Panesar, *Precision Health and Artificial Intelligence*,
https://doi.org/10.1007/978-1-4842-9162-7_5

Responsible Development and Ethical AI Principles

First, the human race will achieve population-level AI-driven precision health only if systems are developed and deployed responsibly. As AI risks continue to grow, so does the number of public and private organizations releasing ethical principles to guide the development and use of AI. Many consider this approach as the most efficient proactive risk mitigation strategy, while a pivotal question remains on whose ethics guidelines are set.

Establishing ethical principles can assist organizations in protecting individual rights and liberties while improving well-being and the common good. Ethicists can translate these principles into norms and practices by organizations, which can then be governed. Many of the guiding principles of AI ethics are principles of biomedical ethics and include reliability and safety, inclusivity, lack of bias, and privacy. Core ethical AI principles fall into two classifications.

- Epistemic principles constitute the prerequisites for investigating AI ethicality and represent the conditions of knowledge that enable organizations to determine whether an AI system is consistent with an ethical code. Principles comprise interpretability, reliability, robustness, and security.

- General ethical AI principles, meanwhile, represent behavioral principles that are valid in many cultural and geographical applications and suggest how AI solutions should behave when faced with moral decisions or dilemmas in a specific field of usage. Principles comprise accountability, data privacy, lawfulness, safety, benevolence, fairness, and human agency.

Epistemic Principles

Both epistemology and ethics are concerned with assessment. Ethics assesses conduct, and epistemology assesses beliefs and cognitive acts. Epistemic principles represent the conditions of knowledge that enable stakeholders to determine whether an AI system is consistent with an ethical principle.

Interpretability

When humans understand the reasoning behind an AI model's predictions and decisions, an AI model is considered interpretable. Many conventional AI models, such as linear regression and decision trees, are simple to understand. In other words, the more interpretable an AI model, the easier it is for someone to understand and trust the computed outputs. The interpretability of a machine learning model refers to how accurately it can associate a cause with an effect. The interpretability of a model is typically affected by its complexity. For example, a linear regression with five features is significantly more interpretable than one with 100 features.

Standard approaches for creating interpretable models are typically outperformed by black boxes, making a trade-off between model accuracy and interpretability. Neural networks are an example of an unexplainable algorithm where output cannot explain the backpropagation algorithm's computed values. Ignorance around constructing AI systems or allowing unexplainable black boxes will lead to problematic eventualities. If an agent were found to be making false predictions, for example, it would be a near-impossible task to rationalize a single behavior that is hidden away and virtually undiscoverable.

In contrast, explainability has to do with the ability of the parameters used within AI models to justify the results.

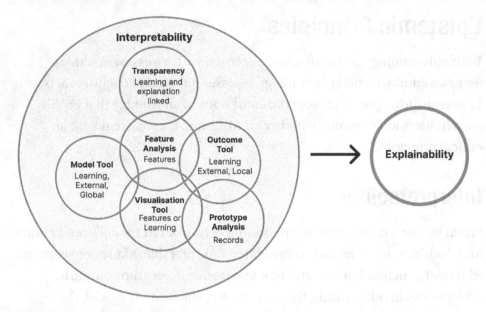

Figure 5-1. *Relationship between interpretability and explainability*

Interpretable, explainable AI facilitates patient-centered care by providing clinicians and patients with the necessary information for shared decision-making. Meaningful conversations about the potential benefits and risks of various courses of action can be supported with data and ensure patients receive treatments best suited to their situation, values, and priorities. One could argue that black-box AI is opposed to the tenets of patient-centered medicine. If clinicians cannot fully comprehend the features and calculations that led to a decision, they can't explain how specific outcomes or recommendations were derived.

Reliability and Safety

Precision health systems must perform reliably, accurately, and safely. Bodies such as the FDA in the United States and MHRA in the United Kingdom promote safety and effectiveness by requiring providers to demonstrate these features. When applied to precision health technologies, ensuring outputs are technically reliable in that AI systems have learned correlations from previously seen data and are clinically reliable is paramount.

Ethicists must also balance patient empowerment against risks such as inconsistent oversight of at-home tests, the importance of clinically supervised care, false positive and negative results, incorrectly reported data, and unintended consequences. AI systems augment current care rather than replace it and may sometimes require human intervention.

Imagine an AI system trained to triage obese patients into high and low risk for heart attack. If the system understood from the data that researchers used to train the model that South Asian patients were less likely to die of a heart attack, it might recommend that South Asian patients are at low risk. However accurate this correlation from the data, the conclusion is a misinterpretation that research clinically contradicts. Being of South Asian ethnicity, in reality, increases your risk of heart and circulatory disease, type 2 diabetes, and a variety of co-morbidities.[1]

Self-improving AI presents another challenge in terms of ensuring reliability and safety. Current regulations assume that products should be clinically tested, manufactured, marketed, and used in a consistent, unchanging form. This is challenging with continuous learning AI, which is constantly changing due to the interpretation and analysis of currently available data. Because of the dynamic nature of continuous learning AI, new methods for ensuring the safety and reliability of such systems will be required. Continuously learning AI requires regulation that provides that ostensible improvements the continuous learning system makes to itself do not instead introduce errors into the model that could cause harm. At the same time, regulation must not require near-constant revalidation of the model.

---

[1] Lobstein, T. and Jackson-Leach, R., 2006. Estimated burden of paediatric obesity and co-morbidities in Europe. Part 2. Numbers of children with indicators of obesity-related disease. International Journal of Pediatric Obesity, 1(1), pp.33–41.

As has been demonstrated with Caucasian-focused medical textbooks used to deliver healthcare education for generations, the evidence base for most genetic tests is limited and needs more data from diverse populations.[2] Diversity and cultural differences play a crucial role in how stakeholders interpret safety in precision health. Until data from under-represented communities is collected at a representative scale, everyone should question it. Clinical tests are helpful only when they provide reliable, actionable information that patients and healthcare professionals can use for clinical decision-making, similar to how behavioral change interventions are beneficial only when they engage people in adopting and maintaining lifestyle behaviors.

At a population level, the interpretation of multi-omics, clinical, environmental, and lifestyle data becomes more complex with inadequate validation of biomarkers and insufficient evidence of clinical utility. The lack of scientific evidence behind individualized precision health solutions is a challenge to safety. For instance, spending money on genomic tests is helpful only if it is beneficial. However, we must anticipate that some new tests will fail to meet expectations. Similarly, individual risk, which is not calculated bespoke to the patient and instead uses established risk prediction models validated on nonrepresentative populations, is counterintuitive to the aims of precision health. However, we must be mindful that supporting the efficacy and tolerability of novel individualized treatments will take time.

Despite best efforts, AI systems cannot provide perfect accuracy due to different errors. Naturally, imperfect datasets may record errors or noise, and random errors are likely to be false positive and false negative predictions.

---

[2] Ioannidis, J.P. and Khoury, M.J., 2018. Evidence-based medicine and big genomic data. Human molecular genetics, 27(R1), pp.R2–R7.

General Ethical AI Principles

General ethical AI principles represent principles that are largely unanimous and valid across cultures and geographies.

Bias, Inclusivity, and Fairness

Any tool used within healthcare, precision or not, should treat everyone fairly and equitably. AI technologies should promote prosperity, preserve solidarity, and avoid unfairness. However, in practice, AI models are not inherently objective. AI models learn the biases that influence human decision-making.[3]

Bias refers to the risk that models may operate in a discriminatory or exclusionary way, and bias can be introduced into a system in many ways. Machine bias can result from several causes, including a developer's discrimination of data used to train the model. Data bias refers to deviation from expected outcomes. Human bias refers to bias exhibited by humans. Without awareness and control, AI systems can amplify existing biases and unfairness within datasets. For instance, research has found that doctors can transmit prejudice under objective descriptions in medical notes.[4]

Clinicians can use something as harmless as a pair of quotation marks to convey bias.[5] When physicians were characterizing their patients' symptoms or health issues, one team of researchers discovered that Black patients, in particular, were quoted in their records more frequently than other patients. Researchers found quotation mark patterns that could

---

[3] Panesar, A. (2021). Machine learning and AI ethics. In Machine Learning and AI for Healthcare (pp. 207-247). Apress, Berkeley, CA.

[4] Sun, M., Oliwa, T., Peek, M. E., & Tung, E. L. (2022). Negative Patient Descriptors: Documenting Racial Bias In The Electronic Health Record: Study examines racial bias in the patient descriptors used in the electronic health record. Health Affairs, 41(2), 203-211.

[5] Beach, M. C., Saha, S., Park, J., Taylor, J., Drew, P., Plank, E., ... & Chee, B. (2021). Testimonial injustice: linguistic bias in the medical records of Black patients and women. Journal of general internal medicine, 36(6), 1708-1714.

signify disrespect, used to communicate irony or sarcasm to future clinical readers. Among the phrases highlighted by the researchers were colloquial language or statements made in Black or ethnic slang.

Ultimately, AI systems reflect the biases inherent in data, those who develop the systems, and clinicians who implement and interpret them. Figure 5-2 details the three aspects of a fair and bias-free AI system.

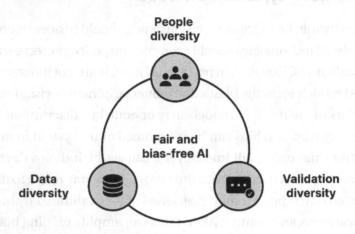

Figure 5-2. *Fair and bias-free AI*

Successful outcomes in precision health rely heavily on the availability of high-quality, high-fidelity data representative of the target patient population. Poorly representative datasets introduce biases, leading to costly misdiagnosis or overdiagnosis scenarios. Only recently, researchers found that AI-powered skin cancer detection apps could better identify events in white patients than patients of other ethnicities. We must do better to ensure equity and equality of precision health access and outcomes.

Representative data can still contain bias because they reflect our society's disparities and intolerances, including racial, geographic, or socioeconomic disparities in healthcare service access. Reliance on data collected via user-facing apps and wearables, for example, may favor socioeconomically advantaged populations with greater access to expensive devices. Similarly, genetic testing remains prohibitively expensive for many consumers, so AI systems that use such genetic datasets may favor more economically advantaged consumers.

Healthcare providers may unfairly implement precision health technologies designed to predict health outcomes and decide who receives care to reduce costs. Ensuring precision health technologies are developed by diverse people, multistakeholder involvement, and discretionary professional judgment will mitigate inequalities in patient-centered care and treatment. Diversity provides a spectrum of thinking, ethics, and mindsets and promotes inclusion, fairness, and representation.

Transparency and Accountability

AI and technology are already influencing people's daily lives. Precision health system decisions will significantly impact patients' health and lifestyle as technologies become more complex and sophisticated. Therefore, individuals engaging with precision health systems must understand how they make decisions. However, transparency goes beyond explaining a system's results. Transparency includes the following:

- Teaching clinicians and patients how to use the results

- Understanding system limitations

- Minimizing undue stress and reliance

As precision health systems become embedded in the prediction and diagnosis of disease and the selection of treatment options, the themes of accountability and liability require attention. Clinicians must understand the clinical justifications behind recommendations from precision health systems. As highlighted, system outputs may be technically relevant but may not always be clinically relevant to a particular individual, so clinicians must exercise their professional discretion. Transparency and accountability are pillars of reliability, fairness, and safety.

Developers of precision health systems must bear proportionate accountability for how systems operate, and providers that deploy systems in clinical practice should exercise consideration when integrating them into clinical practice.

Lawfulness

Legislation and guidelines already minimize many of the risks associated with precision medicine. However, this is an evolving theme. If the benefits of precision medicine are realized, the ethical principle of justice would require universal access to precision medicine for all people. Improvements in patient education must significantly enhance the potential for autonomous patient decisions. In any case, clinicians must use the highest possible level of data security and communication guidelines to avoid harm from test results. Additionally, providers should further examine the cost-effectiveness of precision medicine to prevent malinvestment.

A novel area of lawfulness is the liability of AI systems. Most liability frameworks place the onus on the end-user clinician, provider, or another human who caused harm. With AI, however, errors may occur without any human input at all. Thus, the clinical liability framework requires adjusting accordingly. While providers are responsible for utilizing regulated and demonstrated technologies, deficient liability policies will ultimately prevent patients from realizing the benefits of precision health. Finally, liability for negligence would lie with the person, people, or entities who caused the damage or defect or might have foreseen the product being used in the way that patients used it. Liability needs to be clarified as many parties are involved in AI system development (such as data providers, developers, and the AI system itself), making liability even harder for establishing when something goes wrong.

Data Privacy and Security

According to professionals and patients, the collection of health data carries a high risk of misuse.[6] AI-driven precision health systems should be safe and secure and respect privacy. Data privacy and sharing are critical themes in a precision healthcare model. However, one only has to look at the hacking of global institutions such as Opus, Telus, and Babylon to see that privacy cannot be guaranteed. The biggest hack in history occurred in 2022, when Optus, the Australian communications giant, was compromised by an unsophisticated attack that exposed one in three Australians to potential identity theft and fraud. Within hours, a sample of the data was made available on the dark net.[7]

While data confidentiality is realized through technological advances, people remain suspicious of whether the people entrusted with confidentiality can guarantee data security. Regardless of how intelligent or not systems may be, hackers are only getting smarter.

The willingness to participate in research and provide genetic information, lifestyle, environmental, or medical data also varies. It is also significantly affected by concerns about data security. Research has shown people are highly willing to donate data and participate in real-world and digital trials, but trust in professionals, costs, counseling about test results, and privacy persist. The primary concern isn't just hackers; patients and professionals alike are concerned that genetic data could find its way into the hands of insurance companies and employers, resulting in genetic discrimination. Genetic information must be integrated into electronic

---

[6] Kalkman, S., van Delden, J., Banerjee, A., Tyl, B., Mostert, M. and van Thiel, G., 2022. Patients' and public views and attitudes towards the sharing of health data for research: a narrative review of the empirical evidence. Journal of medical ethics, 48(1), pp.3–13.

[7] Oxford Analytica, 2022. Recovery cost of Optus hack will be huge. Emerald Expert Briefings, (oxan-es).

health records for precision healthcare, making the data even more valuable and vulnerable to cybercriminal attacks.

Data scientists must therefore give data security high priority. Many advise that researchers should limit the collection and linking of genetic, environmental, or lifestyle data to necessary information. However, regulators will only allay stakeholder fears by creating protections for health. Genetic information providers can access and ensure that genetic discrimination is outlawed like it is for sex, disability, and race. Providing penalties for those compromising systems that are proportionate to the acts or crimes committed is vital.

Data sharing is necessary to advance research and develop new tests and therapies. Yet despite its importance, there are many barriers still to overcome. For instance, how much data is too much data? Take religion and spirituality in healthcare, where little attention has been given to the unique context of religion and spirituality and their applicability to precision medicine. Patients' faith is already recognized as a relevant clinical practice consideration to provide more salient and efficacious treatment, particularly in mental health, end-of-life care, and organ donation. Taking into account religious beliefs and practices will most likely result in more effective treatment.

Data sharing has important implications for individual and group privacy and confidentiality. For example, in the context of inherited cancers, is there a clinical duty to warn family members who may develop a particular genetic disease? Because genetic information is confidential to families rather than individuals, clinicians could share information about a genetic disposition with all at-risk family members. Current laws and regulations need to provide a clear answer, with arbitrators coming to inconsistent conclusions regarding a clinician's responsibility to transparency.

Human Agency

Unique ethical issues arise in precision medicine because of the enormous amounts of data generated by clinical whole-genome sequencing, lifestyle and behavioral data, and the extent of current uncertainties concerning data interpretations and disease associations. Among the most ethically challenging issues for clinicians are complicated informed consent processes.

Informed consent is an autonomous, typically written authorization with which the patient gives a doctor permission to perform a medical act. It is one of the most critical safeguards of patients' autonomy. Informed consent is based on comprehensive and understandable information about the nature and risks of a medical procedure and the absence of interference with the patient's voluntary decision to have the procedure performed. There is currently no ethical consensus on whether disclosing the use of an opaque clinical AI algorithm should be a requirement of informed consent. Failure to disclose the use of an obfuscated AI system may jeopardize patients' autonomy and harm the doctor-patient relationship, threatening patients' trust and violating clinical recommendations.

Suppose a patient was to find out in hindsight that a clinician's recommendation was derived from an opaque (i.e., nontransparent) AI system. In that case, this may not only lead the patient to challenge the advice but might also lead to a justified request for an explanation—which the clinician would not be able to provide in the case of an opaque system. Opaque medical AI can thus impede the provision of accurate information, potentially jeopardizing informed consent. As a result, appropriate ethical and explainability standards are required to protect informed consent's autonomy-preserving function.

As we adopt AI technologies and accept their decisions, we acceptingly cede segments of our decision-making to nonhuman systems. This highlights the balance required between autonomy for ourselves and that delegated to artificial agents, affirming the principle of independence within AI.

Beneficence

Beneficence encourages the creation of beneficial AI or AI created for humanitarian benefit ("do good"). At the same time, nonmaleficence refers to AI's negative consequences and risks ("no harm"). Beneficence is essential because it ensures that the principle of AI technology is to promote well-being, preserve dignity, and sustain the planet.

Generally, AI ethics have been primarily concerned with the principle of nonmaleficence; negative consequences must be avoided, for example, misclassification. Beneficence can be understood through evaluating the probability and magnitude of potential harms to participants, assessment of risks, and mitigation strategies against possible benefits to the individual, people represented by participants, and society.

Redesigning Care and the Patient-Clinician Relationship

Precision health is changing the way care is delivered and with it the patient-clinician relationship. Genomics research and approaches leveraging big data, whether electronic medical records or large-scale health tracking, are reorientating the clinical experience from prevention through to diagnosis and treatment as an increasingly comprehensive vision of personalized medicine is realized.

Rather than being dichotomously sick or healthy, precision health replaces a taxonomy of diseases with a multilayer characterization of individuals.

Take the example of patients waiting within traditional care when a screening test presents an abnormal finding but is uncertain whether and when the individual will develop the condition. When diagnosed, patients move to treatment, whereas within precision health individuals are closely monitored and given care through the continuum. Health data will enable the quantification of risk factors for particular diseases, allow for the customization of care, and determine deterioration, morbidity, and mortality risks. Care spans past biomarkers and how people biologically differ to include how and where people spend their time and the obstacles in making health-promoting decisions.

Hospital care is moving outside of the care ward. Virtual wards provide wrap-around care to people in their own homes to reduce the need for a hospital admission. For a person with complex health conditions, a virtual community is about better self-care, self-awareness, and confidence to handle standard flare-ups at home. For doctors caring for complex patients at risk from hospital admissions, the virtual ward provides "extra backup" and hands-on support by monitoring patients daily to see where the action is required, often saving valuable time and duplication for the clinical teams.

The core virtual ward mimics a typical hospital setup. It includes a ward coordinator, a doctor, a district nurse (DN), a community matron, a practice nurse (PN), and a practice administrator. Local community support workers (CSW) and advocacy workers are also invited to attend. Depending on local health needs, therapists, a community geriatrician, or other healthcare professionals could prove invaluable team members. Read more about Gro Health, a multiplatform system that provides a stellar example of a virtual ward implemented to good effect. Figure 5-3 shows an example of a virtual ward.

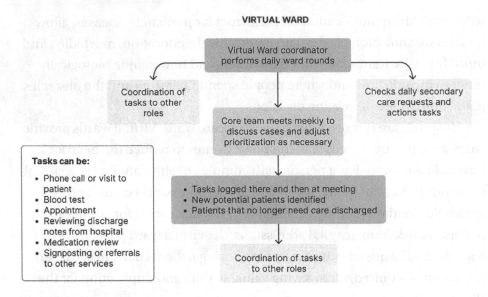

VIRTUAL WARD

Virtual Ward coordinator performs daily ward rounds

Coordination of tasks to other roles

Checks daily secondary care requests and actions tasks

Core team meets meekly to discuss cases and adjust prioritization as necessary

Tasks can be:
- Phone call or visit to patient
- Blood test
- Appointment
- Reviewing discharge notes from hospital
- Medication review
- Signposting or referrals to other services

- Tasks logged there and then at meeting
- New potential patients identified
- Patients that no longer need care discharged

Coordination of tasks to other roles

Figure 5-3. *A virtual ward*

With healthcare professionals in short supply, it is doubtful that practitioners will feel threatened by AI regarding loss of authority and autonomy. Paradoxically, the burden of uncertainty innate in a probabilistic diagnosis increases the expectation that the supposedly precise diagnosis will empower patients by enabling better-informed decisions about future treatments. Depending on socioeconomic status, culture, age, and psychological disposition, patients may differ in their ability to manage this tension. As the patient-clinician relationship evolves, researchers must investigate the impact of precision health and quality of life.

Health Inequalities

While precision health aims to improve outcomes at both patient and population health levels, we must ensure advances in science and technology do not worsen health inequalities. Minority communities frequently face discrimination in healthcare and receive poor medical treatment across the globe. Outreach to minority communities—especially in the research field—has also been characterized by a long history of exploitation, abuse, and marginalization.

Factors contributing to health inequalities include cost, access, and under-representation. Cost is a prohibitive factor that makes technologies accessible to those who can afford them. Many payers may not reimburse some new services, limiting care provision to those who can afford it. Failure to address systemic bias in data provision and genetic databases will only worsen disparities.

Theology

Genetic exploration, whether IVF, genetic engineering, or gene therapy, has raised questions of morality for religious and spiritual communities. Within years, human brains will interface with computers, nanotechnologies will be embedded within human tissue, 3D organs will be printed and transplanted, and people will select optimal embryos to minimize the potential of severe or life-limiting diseases in their offspring. The theological and philosophical challenges of precision health are imperative to developing rigorous clinical practices and associated laws.

Preparing the Profession

The advancement of AI-powered precision health technologies has raised concerns about whether these systems will eventually replace doctors. Such situations are most likely unfounded. Most, if not all, countries face severe clinician shortages, which are expected to worsen over the next decade. For example, a report for the Association of American Medical Colleges predicts a physician shortage through 2030 under every scenario modeled. Rather than posing a threat to clinicians, AI-infused precision health tools are critical to improving care efficiency and mitigating some of the concerns that will arise due to future shortages of trained and experienced clinicians.[8, 9] Further still, augmenting clinicians with digital transformation and implementation support would propel adoption of AI-powered technologies further.

The promise of precision health systems to improve care likely will come not from replacing clinicians but rather in automating repetitive tasks, thereby freeing clinicians time to focus on high-value activities in the patient care and treatment process. In this regard, properly designed systems will focus on augmenting the skills and experience of highly trained clinicians in keeping with the natural workflows of clinical delivery processes.

Summary

As precision health is realized and digital devices, data, and AI play an increasingly important part in our day-to-day lives, the most important question will become whether and under which conditions precision health can improve patients' quality of life.

Quality of life is adjudged by patients themselves as being good or as subjectively worse due to over-compliance and engagement with the constant behavioral aspects of one's health.

---

[8] Baptiste, D.L., Commodore-Mensah, Y., Alexander, K.A., Jacques, K., Wilson, P.R., Akomah, J., Sharps, P. and Cooper, L.A., 2020. COVID-19: Shedding light on racial and health inequities in the USA. Journal of clinical nursing.

[9] Barnett, M.L., Luis Sanchez, B.E., Green Rosas, Y. and Broder-Fingert, S., 2021. Future directions in lay health worker involvement in children's mental health services in the US. Journal of Clinical Child & Adolescent Psychology, 50(6), pp.966–978.

CHAPTER 6

Future of Precision Healthcare

Digital health technologies and AI are already creating intelligent processes and workflows that make healthcare delivery cheaper, more effective, personalized, and more equitable. Yet precision health seeks to go beyond this and improve patient management and diagnoses by understanding the human condition and experience deeper. Much of the emphasis has been placed on the potential for developing better medicines based on an increased understanding of disease pathology. Now that data and technology are readily available and affordable, improvements in diagnostics and support are enabling better patient management. The quantity and complexity of data reflect a patient's genetics, environment, and lifestyle.

Big data and AI technologies provide enormous potential to identify new conditions and prognostic indicators, provide precision behavioral change support, and rehabilitation or identify patients who will respond better to treatments. Yet this is not without its challenges.

The greater the level of detail with which we understand patients, the greater the demand for information management, accountability, and transparency. And while we develop more profound knowledge about delivering personalized care, how do we use this knowledge to reduce the incidence of future disease and mitigate the technical, clinical, and ethical issues that arise? Should precision medicine prioritize prevention over cure, which is much the focus of current medicine? Do you want to know that you are at risk of developing a disease if there is no treatment or cure for it? There are many issues to consider when dealing with technologies that predict future possibilities of unknown magnitude and significance. This chapter identifies important themes in pursuing precision health and posits potential impact and consequence.

Precision Care from Birth to Death

Low-cost genetic testing provides a human gene map that clinicians can use to understand an individual's health and disposition to disease. Targeted next-generation sequencing enables rapid identification of common and rare genetic variations. Detecting variants contributing to therapeutic drug response or adverse effects is essential for implementing individualized pharmacotherapy and provision of support. Rather than behavioral support delivered as an intervention, lifestyle support will be provided from birth through digital therapeutics alongside prescribed pharmacological interventions that will one day be supported by nanotechnologies to offer therapy and support and replenish the body. Clinicians, supported by automated technologies, will analyze the state of health and disease risk in real time. As each person receives more significant access to richer, real-time, granular data about themselves, they will learn more about themselves and, if this information is made public, about others in the community. It is feasible that given population-level genetic, lifestyle, and behavioral data, AI may not just predict ill health and disease but also approximate the exact point of death. Figure 6-1 shows inputs and outputs of a precision healthcare tool.

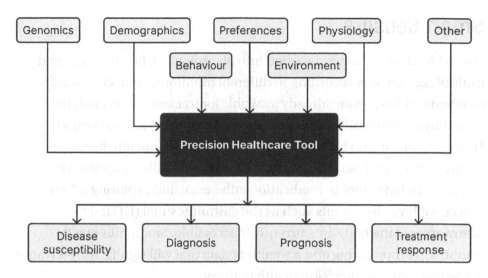

Figure 6-1. *Precision healthcare tool: inputs and outputs*

Nanotechnology

A nanometer is one-billionth of a meter (0.000000001 m), which amounts to the width of three to five atoms. Nanobots are currently around 0.1–10 micrometers in diameter, so they are not quite at the nano scale. However, nanobots can be used, for instance, to perform chemotherapy precisely on cancer cells. Nanobot delivery would decrease the negative effect of chemotherapy on healthy cells and improve patient health and well-being.

DNA Manipulation and Gene Therapy

Gene therapy, the treatment of disease through the manipulation of DNA, is one of the fastest-growing areas of precision health, with more than 2,000 therapies in development across the world. It is hoped that researchers can find cures for infectious and noncommunicable diseases by making precise changes to the human genome. Concerns remain, however, that poorer countries lacking infrastructure for manufacturing and delivering gene therapy by default lack access to such treatments.

Smart Sensors

Wearable sensors can be classified into physiological, biochemical, and multiplexed sensors according to different monitoring objects. Wearable biochemical sensors are already available for tracking target analytes in readily available biological fluids (such as saliva, tears, and sweat). However, sensors are becoming smaller and even more intelligent. Smart pills are such an example—small ingestible pills equipped with sensors that have roles in medication adherence and exploring otherwise inaccessible environments such as the gastrointestinal (GI) tract. Many areas of the body are currently inaccessible. Smart pills enable unobtrusive monitoring and a wealth of data that will significantly advance understanding and precision health delivery.

Bioprinting

Bioprinting will revolutionize medicine as we know it. N, not only because delivering new organs and live material to where it is needed is time-sensitive and crucial but because there needs to be more of them. Additionally, the recipient's immune system can reject donated organs, causing the donor organ to fail.

3D printing is already used to customize body parts such as knee implants. 3D printing creates a three-dimensional object by reading a digital blueprint and reproducing successive layers using filament and ultraviolet light. While entire organs still haven't been developed, bioprinting has enabled mini-organs on a chip, equating to tiny cell samples of tissue that mimic the functions and structures of their full-grown counterparts. The laboratory-grown mini organs allow pharmaceutical companies to test drugs on versions of human tissue and assess their effectiveness or toxicity instead of using unreliable and ethically problematic animal models.

Bioprinted organs further progress precision care as they are made from an individual's tissue, ensuring that they are customized for each body. Customization minimizes the chances that the host's body will reject the organ, meaning the organ will last longer and won't need treatment for complications such as rejection. Bioprinting will replace dysfunctional biostructures, whether at 6 months or 60 years old. Ethical issues surrounding bioprinting include equal access to treatment, clinical safety complications, and the enhancement of the human body.

Brain Computer Interfacing

As we age, healthy older adults may have difficulties communicating, concentrating, memorizing, talking, walking, or maintaining balance.[1] These symptoms may also be experienced by elderly patients and can lead to the inability to communicate with family, climb stairs, remember new information, or drive safely. For example, most older people need to use assistive technologies to perform daily-life activities better, such as increasing the zoom of a display or using handrails to get upstairs. To compound matters, the aging process does not affect people uniformly.

Many patients with cognitive or physical impairments are now being treated with brain-computer interface technology. As a promising and growing technology for assisting and improving communication/control, brain-computer interfaces are becoming increasingly popular among people with motor paralysis (paraplegia and quadriplegia) as a result of stroke, cerebral palsy, and amyotrophic lateral sclerosis (ALS).

This technology promises to significantly enhance patients' quality of life by considerably improving their autonomy and mobility. It is possible to use a brain-computer interface (BCI) as an assistive, adaptive, and

---

[1] Belkacem, A.N., Jamil, N., Palmer, J.A., Ouhbi, S. and Chen, C., 2020. Brain computer interfaces for improving the quality of life of older adults and elderly patients. Frontiers in Neuroscience, 14, p.692.

rehabilitation technology to monitor brain activity and translate specific signals that reveal the elderly's intent into commands. BCI systems could be helpful for older adults in many ways, such as training their motor/cognitive abilities to prevent aging effects, controlling home appliances, communicating with others during daily activities, and controlling an exoskeleton to enhance the strength of the body's joints.

Brain-computer technology has clinical and nonclinical applications in many areas, including medicine, entertainment, education, and psychology, to solve many health issues, such as cognitive deficits, slowness in processing speed, impaired memory, and movement capability decline among older adults, which can affect the quality of elderly life and adversely affect mental health.

Smart Habitats

In recent years, cities worldwide, as well as less urbanized areas and the countryside, have begun to become "smart" in many ways due to the Internet of Things (IoT) and its core and complementary technologies. The IoT is made of sensors and other components that connect our version of the world made of atoms (i.e., us humans, our body systems/health, and our devices, vehicles, roads, buildings, plants, animals, etc.) with a digital mirror version made of bits. This link enables cities and regions, both urban and rural, to be self-aware and agile in near real time, based on changes in populations and environments that are continuously monitored and captured by sensors, similar to how a living being's internal biological systems operate and respond to their environment. Big data collected by various IoT sensors can also be used to forecast the near future with reasonable accuracy, allowing for better planned responses/mitigation.

Sensors embedded into physical environments collecting continuous data in ambient intelligent environments can look for changes in health status and provide in-the-home health interventions. By gaining real-time access to this information, city services can respond promptly to urgent health needs and make decisions to avoid unhealthy situations. Depending upon the device used, sensors can collect additional information. Many devices have cameras and microphones that provide a dense data source indicative of the user's state and environment. Use of other apps on devices, including phone calls and texting, can also be captured.

Smart homes offer tremendous benefits for health monitoring and intervention; however, they remain at risk for cyberattacks. This new type of criminality may obtain details about inhabitants' living patterns, putting the residents' safety at risk. Other forms of security risk may rise even when there is no malicious intent. For example, health monitoring devices that do not follow prescribed software standards can endanger lives by not providing critical information at the needed time.

The intention is to live healthier and happier lives because of, and within, smart habitats. However, the COVID pandemic showed that authorities can use data and digital technologies to enforce rules and regimes that may oppose ethical consensus or widespread agreement. During the COVID lockdowns in the UAE, for instance, people were allowed to visit public places only if they could show proof of vaccination.[2]

Autonomous technologies will transform cars into more than just a means of transport. Apart from the fundamental premise that autonomous vehicles will take over driving responsibilities, the more significant leap is that transport will free riders to explore the potential to improve their body, mind, and environment. What's more, health and well-being in transportation are required to achieve a zero-accident future, for example, through early detection of ailments and assistance in emergencies. At its very basic, a connected vehicle can send SOS notifications, connect to the emergency services in case of an accident, or adjust a seat to

---

[2] Khan, M.L., Malik, A., Ruhi, U. and Al-Busaidi, A., 2022. Conflicting attitudes: Analyzing social media data to understand the early discourse on COVID-19 passports. Technology in Society, 68, p.101830.

accommodate the best posture. Location services will provide allergen warnings, and biosensors that enable monitoring of blood alcohol, blood pressure, and heart rate could provide features such as drunk-driving prevention and an indication of drowsiness.

Collaboration is the bedrock of change, and this is especially true when it comes to realizing precision healthcare. To provide tailored care for everyone, robust collaboration and synergistic efforts involving multiple stakeholders are essential.

Digital Health Education

For some people, the digital transformation that the COVID pandemic brought was a blessing; for others, it was very much a curse. More people and environments have become digitally connected, with local authorities, charities, and governments even providing mobile devices and mobile data for those who need it. Health app use rose sharply, too, as patients sought to self-manage their health. Patient management grew from health apps to providing remote consultations and digital health solutions. While attitudes were primarily influenced by digital literacy, accessibility, and training, which appear to be linked with age, whichever way the public understood it, there is no doubt this highlighted the need for up-to-date digital health education.

Despite the lack of a formal definition of digital health, acceptable suggestions, such as those provided by the Food and Drug Administration, include classifications such as health information technology, wearable devices, telehealth and telemedicine, personalized medicine, and general wellness. Table 6-1 lists the areas of digital health education.

Table 6-1. *Areas of Digital Health Education*

Theme	Description
Digital therapeutics	Software (mobile, web, other) that provides evidence-based intervention meeting the definition of a medical device, including precision behavioral health intervention.
Telehealth	Telecommunications and digital communication technologies are used to deliver and facilitate health and health-related services such as medical treatment, provider and patient education, health information services, and self-care.
Wearable devices and sensors	Wearable electronics are devices that can be worn or bonded with human skin to continually and carefully monitor a person's actions without interfering with or limiting the user's movement.
Digital biomarkers	Measurement of physiological data in real time using hardware and software for prognostic or diagnostic purposes.

In this context, digital health education is specifically designed to transfer an understanding of the practical use of digital technologies, including health apps, artificial intelligence, and wearables within healthcare systems, to healthcare professionals. Digital health education is vital for many reasons, but none more so than to bridge the gap between what is expected by patients and the teaching of healthcare staff or students to enable implementation and realize the benefits of digital healthcare.

Literacy

A generational shift is underway. The millennial generation is now past, and Generation Z is leaving high school and entering higher education. Generation Z is typically digitally native, accepting of the use of technology in their lives while not necessarily being well-versed in how to use it.

Generations X and Y generally are less digitally savvy and form a significant part of the health workforce. Research has shown that older people usually have more substantial training needs regarding digital literacy.[3]

Digital health education is necessary to ensure digital literacy among new and incumbent healthcare workers so that they can fully utilize the tools at their disposal. For example, a clinician would not need to know all of the diabetes digital therapeutics available for mobile phones but would be able to assess an individual patient's needs, such as clinical history and digital literacy, to make an actionable recommendation to patients.

Clinicians must learn how to work with data-enabled technology applications and develop knowledge and skills to use precision health tools in healthcare delivery. It becomes impossible for a physician to bear all the data management and analysis responsibilities, not to mention patient communications. The application of AI in healthcare aims to advise clinicians with better and faster insights to improve patients' lives ultimately. It will be necessary for healthcare professionals to be able to use and interpret information from these technologies and be equipped to deal with any potential challenges that may arise.

Healthcare providers are slowly realizing that adopting multiple digital platforms is inefficient and costly. Many healthcare networks have invested in digital platforms that provide various services or interventions (for instance, virtual wards or weight management, cardiac rehabilitation, and diabetes services). Using a single or a minimal number of platforms that provides remote patient monitoring and data analytics across health areas minimizes the resources required to deploy successful technologies. Precision medicine relies on an increasing amount of heterogeneous data of molecular genetics, clinical, and biological parameters for each

---

[3] Martínez-Alcalá, C.I., Rosales-Lagarde, A., Alonso-Lavernia, M.D.L.Á., Ramírez-Salvador, J.Á., Jiménez-Rodríguez, B., Cepeda-Rebollar, R.M., López-Noguerola, J.S., Bautista-Díaz, M.L. and Agis-Juárez, R.A., 2018. Digital inclusion in older adults: A comparison between face-to-face and blended digital literacy workshops. Frontiers in ICT, 5, p.21.

patient, with the total number of parameters for medical decision-making on a single patient estimated to be up to 10,000. Using as few systems as possible enables providers to realize associated benefits such as scalable efficiencies in staff training, upskilling, implementation, and deployment costs.

Improving digital literacy among healthcare workers also enhances their interest in digital technologies. While this may not appear to be an essential aspect of digital health education, clinician apathy and enthusiasm can directly affect patient engagement with digital health technologies. Research has shown that clinical apathy toward digital health technologies can affect a patient's engagement.[4]

Changing Roles

The paternalistic clinician-patient relationship has been transformed into an equal partnership with shared medical decision-making. Digitization of healthcare has provided access to big-data information and cognitive insights to caregivers and patients, transforming healthcare and clinical workflows. The point of care has shifted from the clinic and physician to the patient.

Experience-based medicine has evolved into evidence-based and patient-centered approaches. Clinicians require education on the changing role of healthcare professionals and how digital health technologies can support more tailored patient-centered care and clinical decision-making and relieve repetitive tasks enabling more focus on other aspects of patient care. As we move to the age of precision health, digital health education will provide knowledge of information platforms and intelligence tools in healthcare and the skills to use them effectively.

---

[4] Slevin, P., Kessie, T., Cullen, J., Butler, M.W., Donnelly, S.C. and Caulfield, B., 2019. Exploring the potential benefits of digital health technology for the management of COPD: a qualitative study of patient perceptions. ERJ open research, 5(2).

A testament to this is the changing role of pharmacists who now provide management tools, facilitate access to care, and provide interventions to extensive populations, including patients with hypertension, hyperlipidemia, diabetes, and cancer.

Quality

Evidence to demonstrate the impact and outcomes of precision health technologies is paramount. There are hundreds of thousands of digital health technologies, and new technologies will continue to emerge and fade in both research and practice. Similarly, most health apps need to reach regulatory standards.[5] Digital health education will focus on frameworks for technology selection and teach learners to identify and evaluate novel, innovative, impactful technologies.

Ability

New aspects of clinical care require formal pedagogy. Patient interactions and e-professionalism must be taught and evaluated alongside other skills as they are fundamental to digital health. Digital health skills include appropriate body language and effective patient communication through virtual interactions. Similarly, to fulfill the adage of doing no harm, clinicians must be sufficiently trained in digital health use, data management, and awareness of technical and clinical risks. Hazards include data and automation biases, where data and algorithms may mirror human biases in decision-making and lack of decision validation.

---

[5] Tarricone, R., Petracca, F., Cucciniello, M. and Ciani, O., 2022. Recommendations for developing a lifecycle, multidimensional assessment framework for mobile medical apps. Health Economics.

Accessibility and Equity

A benefit of digital healthcare is that much of it is cloud-enabled. Enabling learners to understand how the cloud-based nature of communication facilitates accessibility will promote greater accessibility of health interventions for patients. For instance, a cardiac surgeon in Melbourne, Australia, could perform open-heart surgery on a patient in a remote hospital in Guam through the use of telecommunications, robotics, and the support of a facilitator at the scene. Precision health solutions that are accessible and impactful have a tremendous opportunity to foster health equity and achieve health promotion, prevention, and self-care.

Training workforces to understand and use digital health technologies is critical to precision health's success. Importantly, training could democratize skills and knowledge among healthcare teams. However, training is costly as no formal training processes currently exist. Better still, building digital health into university curricula would allow learners to better grasp digital health at large and understand the implications for clinical practice on graduation instead of a snapshot approach, which is limited in learning.

New Forms of Training

An aging population, chronic underfunding in staff development and retention, and the fallout from the COVID-19 pandemic (including the Great Resignation) have left many health systems facing healthcare worker shortages. In the United Kingdom, the NHS has declared a staffing crisis with more than 100,000 job vacancies, the United States is estimated to need 275,000 extra nurses by 2030, and Australia is predicted to have a nursing shortage of 123,000 by the same time.[6, 7, 8] The need for well-trained and qualified healthcare and social workers has never been greater.

However, educating and training professionals to work in health and social care settings is complex and nuanced. Training and professional development for some staff groups are already scarce, and measures to control COVID infection rates contributed to a significant decline in face-to-face exposure to all aspects of training and experiences, creating additional barriers for educators.

Immersive technology is a set of interfaces, applications, and software that create augmented simulations for experiences and perfect interactions between human beings and technology. These include virtual reality (VR), augmented reality (AR), mixed reality (MR), and 360° videos. In virtual reality, the user's reality is replaced by an immersive, entirely digital environment; augmented reality (AR) overlays a digital or 3D environment in the form of objects, vide', or data into the user's environment; and mixed reality (MR) blends both physical and virtual environments.

VR and AR are widespread; however, the hardware and development costs remain high. In contrast, mixed reality uses practical tools for realization, such as 360° videos. As the name suggests, 360° videos consist of video recordings made with a device able to simultaneously capture and combine scenes in a 360°-degree perspective and can be used with head-mounted hardware or on many mobile devices, which significantly

---

[6] The Kings Fund (2022). NHS workforce: our position. [online] The King's Fund. Available at: https://www.kingsfund.org.uk/projects/positions/nhs-workforce.

[7] US Department of Labor announces $80M funding opportunity to help train, expand, diversify nursing workforce; address shortage of nurses | U.S. Department of Labor. [online] Available at: https://www.dol.gov/newsroom/releases/eta/eta20221003.

[8] MacDonald, L. and Stayner, G. (2022). Hospital nurse Julie-Marie has worked in the industry for 20 years, but is thinking about quitting — and she's not alone. ABC News. [online] 21 Jul. Available at: https://www.abc.net.au/news/2022-07-22/nursing-shortage-on-the-cards-due-to-pandemic/101253058.

enhances accessibility and scalability. The viewer can control and change the viewing angle at any stage through head movement. However, 360° videos typically lack some interactivity when compared to VR.

Immersive technology has been shown to improve students' understanding of learning material, learning experience, and knowledge retention and enable on-location virtual simulations that educators cannot teach in a traditional classroom setting. One study found a 230 percent improvement in knowledge retention when comparing immersive technology to traditional face-to-face teaching.[9] Immersive technologies lend themselves perfectly to educating patients and training future workforces. Importantly, immersive technologies provide invaluable experience of simulated events, ensuring confidence, skills, and knowledge. For instance, educators could teach social workers about caring for vulnerable people through simulation, similar to how an aspiring open-heart surgeon could learn to deal with the stress and pressure of a situation by being virtually present in the same room. Immersive technologies will support the training of more people to a better standard than face-to-face learning in a shorter time. The technology also helps healthcare workers to make fewer mistakes through simulation-based learning and data analytics to analyze one's habits, behaviors, and responses within the simulation.

Collaboration Between Academia and Industry

Digital health remains a growing and challenging public health practice, and research methods still need to catch up with the pace of innovation. Digital health end-user engagement remains complex, demanding personalization and adaptive interventions that meet the needs of diverse populations.

---

[9] Young, A. and Aquilina, A., 2021. Use of virtual reality to support rapid upskilling of healthcare professionals during COVID-19 pandemic. In XR Case Studies (pp.137–145). Springer, Cham.

Less meaningful evidence and a lack of understanding of the efficacy and quality of digital health solutions have coerced academics and industry to partner. Academic-industry collaboration (AIC) offers a mechanism to bring disparate sectors together to alleviate digital health challenges of engagement, reach, sustainability, dissemination, evaluation, and equity.

Educators, typically academic institutions or government-affiliated departments, are already partnering with digital health companies to teach about digital health and respond to the requirement for a deep understanding of digital health alongside the clinical curriculum.

Despite the ongoing endorsements for transdisciplinary collaborations in digital health, a limited understanding of successful collaborations exists. Among ethical skepticism toward collaboration, barriers to collaboration include the initiation, maintenance, and sustainment of relationships. There are growing examples of successful collaboration between academia and industry in the digital health marketplace. Chapter 7 contains a case study of a successful partnership between a hospital network and a digital therapeutics provider.

Summary

The future of precision health rests on integrating the abundant technologies that lie before us and the knowledge and skills to use them in clinical practice. As hybrid care becomes more commonplace, so does the requirement not to lose the human touch. Collaborative academic research, clinical evidence, and policymaking must shape the domain of precision healthcare to ensure humanity's best interests are protected. While future possibilities are constrained only by the technologies, devices, and data available, ethically implementing precision healthcare requires careful attention to validation, data interpretation, and protection of data privacy and security.

CHAPTER 7

Precision Healthcare in Practice

Though varied in its implementation across fields, precision medicine has raised hopes of revolutionary treatments and has spurred the proliferation of novel therapeutics and the reconfiguration of healthcare. This chapter will illustrate some of the compelling and temporal complexities of precision health analyzed here under its emerging rubrics.

Health technologies must ultimately do no harm. The determination of patient risk can hence categorize digital technologies. Systems can improve system efficiencies while providing no measurable benefit to patients, inform and provide remote monitoring, encourage behavior change and self-management, provide clinical decision and prediction support to guide treatment, and provide output from which tools can compute and diagnose. However, because regulators' evidentiary requirements are defined by intended use, many digital inventions slip outside of regulation.

Randomized controlled trials (RCTs) are deemed the most powerful and reliable form of evidence for assessing the efficacy of a treatment. Evidence demonstrates that many factors can influence the reliability of RCTs, including methodological quality, reporting quality, and source of funding. Real-world evaluation, or the power of N=1 at scale, disrupts traditional hierarchies and approaches. Disruption can be beneficial

© Arjun Panesar 2023
A. Panesar, *Precision Health and Artificial Intelligence*,
https://doi.org/10.1007/978-1-4842-9162-7_7

because real-world data, in principle, can capture the experience of the majority of people using services rather than the 5–10 percent percent who take part in trials.

The datafication of the human experience through mobile phones, social media, digital communities, health apps, nutrition tracking, wearables, and health IoT has empowered patients to become their own evidence base and influence healthcare academia and understanding.

The pandemic catalyzed healthcare providers to reach for digital tools and scalable technology. Healthcare providers were observed to have differing acceptance thresholds for innovation and could be classified into the typical five archetypes of innovators. However, determining the legitimacy and safety of a new solution is a significant barrier for end users, whether patients or clinicians. Similarly, innovators need to demonstrate benefits and compliance with standards. Unclear end-user expectations, evidence requirements, and an ever-changing regulatory environment are only a few of the challenges in the precision health ecosystem.

The purpose of each case study is to showcase real-world demonstrations of intelligent precision health systems that are innovative and showcase the power and impact of tailored, individualized care.

Fundamental principles and best practices are highlighted with the following case studies:

- "Delivery of Specialist Multidisciplinary Weight Management to Hospital-Based Patients"

- "Understanding People's Attitudes Toward Data for the Optimization of a Specialist Podiatry Service for People with Long-Term Health Conditions"

- "Evaluation of a Digital Intervention for the Self-Management of Type 2 Diabetes and Prediabetes"

- "Voice-Based Symptom Monitoring and AI-Based Rehabilitation for Patients with Long COVID"

- "Supporting Children and Young People to Lead Healthier Lives with Family-Based Behavioral Change Support"

Delivery of Specialist Multidisciplinary Weight Management to Hospital-Based Patients Through a Digital Tool

The following case study presents an example of a precision health tool used within hospitals to deliver multidisciplinary specialist weight management, remote monitoring, and bidirectional communication to facilitate an engaged and collaborative patient-centered ecosystem.

In the United Kingdom, 27 percent of men and 30 percent of women live with obesity[1] and have an increased risk of chronic diseases such as type 2 diabetes (T2D), mental health problems, particular malignancies, and a reduced life expectancy.[2] Moreover, people living with obesity have a greater risk of hospitalization and adverse outcomes (including mortality) from COVID-19.[3] Within the United Kingdom alone, the estimated healthcare cost of obesity management was £6.1 billion (US $8.5 billion)

---

[1] Statistics on Obesity, Physical Activity, and Diet, England, 2019.: NHS England; 2019 Aug 8. https://tinyurl.com/asjjj4yr [accessed 2021-03-03]

[2] Peeters A, Barendregt JJ, Willekens F, Mackenbach JP, Al Mamun A, Bonneux L, NEDCOM, the Netherlands Epidemiology and Demography Compression of Morbidity Research Group. Obesity in adulthood and its consequences for life expectancy: a life-table analysis. Ann Intern Med 2003 Jan 07;138(1):24–32.

[3] Excess weight and COVID-19. Insights from new evidence.: Public Health England. https://tinyurl.com/y4mr8d8e [accessed 2021-11-08]

in 2014—projected to reach £9.7 billion (US $13.5 billion) by 2050—with the broader costs to society estimated at £49.9 billion (US $69.2 billion) per annum.[4]

Within the British-based National Health Service (NHS), a tiered framework underlies the pyramidal structure of obesity management, in which the progressively restricted resources and numbers of patients typify upward tier progression. Obesity management within a primary care setting (tier 1) consists of promoting healthy lifestyles, education, and preventive strategies. Community-based services (tier 2) usually comprise dietary advice and optimized physical activity. For people with more severe obesity (BMI > 40 kg/m2 or BMI > 35 kg/m2 with obesity-related comorbidities), there is hospital-based obesity management (tier 3), which usually consists of a multidisciplinary team, with specialist dieticians, medical staff, and psychological support. Bariatric surgery (tier 4) sits at the top of the structure and as such represents a restricted resource (despite representing an excellent treatment choice for obesity) available to a very small proportion of the obese population who are potentially eligible for this procedure.[5]

Hospital-based management of obesity (within tiers 3 and 4) is restricted and as such does not represent a scalable model applicable to a population level.[6] Furthermore, the demand for obesity services including referrals has augmented in recent years. We illustrate this with the example

---

[4] Health matters: obesity and the food environment.: Public Health England. https://www.gov.uk/government/publications/health-matters-obesity-and-the-food-environment/health-matters-obesity-and-the-food-environment--2 [accessed 2021-03-03]

[5] Obesity: Clinical Assessment and Management (Quality Standard QS127).: NICE https://www.nice.org.uk/guidance/qs127/resources/obesity-clinical-assessment-and-management-pdf-75545363615173 [accessed 2021-02-22]

[6] Supporting weight management services during the COVID-19 pandemic: Phase 1 insights.: Public Health England https://assets.publishing.service.gov.uk/government/uploads/system/uploads/attachment_data/file/915274/WMS_Report.pdf [accessed 2021-02-22]

of our own hospital-based tier 3 and 4 obesity service at University Hospitals Coventry and Warwickshire (UHCW), United Kingdom, with a greater than sixfold increase in the number of referrals over a 5-year period between 2014 (207 new referrals) and 2019 (1,319 new referrals), and more than 1,800 patients currently accessing our obesity service. Despite this surge in new referrals, this number is likely an order of magnitude lower than that of local adults who are eligible for referral to our service, with an estimated 2 percent of men and 4 percent of women currently living in the Coventry and Warwickshire regions who have a BMI greater than 40 kg/m2.[7, 8, 9] Thus, there is a large unmet need for the vast majority of people living with severe obesity in the United Kingdom, for whom the current hospital-based tier 3 and 4 services within the NHS obesity management framework simply fail to deliver. Furthermore, there is often a disjointed patient pathway between the various obesity management tiers within primary, community-based, and secondary care settings. Unfortunately, the COVID-19 pandemic has stymied the effective implementation of obesity management across all tiers, with multiple factors implicated including staff redeployments, repurposing of clinical areas, restrictions of elective procedures, lockdown measures, remote appointments, and patient-based fears that include attendance at healthcare settings.

Digital tools have a huge potential to transform weight management services. Despite the potential utility of various apps for digital and mobile devices within hospital-based tier 3 and 4 obesity management settings, to date such an innovation has not occurred. There is emerging evidence

---

[7] Warwickshire at Glance.: Warwickshire County Council https://api.warwickshire.gov.uk/documents/WCCC-1014-120 [accessed 2021-10-12]

[8] Coventry's population estimate 2018. Coventry City Council. 2018 Jun 1. https://www.coventry.gov.uk/download/downloads/id/27490/coventrys_population_estimate_2018.pdf [accessed 2021-03-04]

[9] Craig S, Conolly A. Health Survey for England 2018: Overweight and obesity in adults and children. NHS Digital. 2018 Nov 1. http://healthsurvey.hscic.gov.uk/media/81625/HSE18-Adult-Child-Obesity-rep.pdf [accessed 2021-03-01]

for the effectiveness of digital tools in the management of obesity. Current evidence shows emerging effectiveness of digital health interventions for specialist weight loss, yet poor uptake and engagement with digital tools remain common challenges with digital health interventions.[10]

Objective

The aim of our study was to assess the feasibility and effectiveness of the Low Carb Program app for weight loss, applied within our specialist hospital-based (tier 3) obesity service. Because of the disrupting effects of the COVID-19 pandemic on our obesity service, we also compared the clinical outcomes from the Low Carb Program app applied in the context of remote patient appointments over the telephone with the prepandemic, traditional standard of care.

Methods

Access to the Low Carb Program app was offered to all new patients at their initial medical consultation after being referred to our hospital-based (tier 3) obesity service at UHCW, United Kingdom, over a 9-month period between January 2020 and September 2020. The initial contact was with a medical doctor. Patients were informed about the app, and those who wanted to use the app were given instructions on how to download it. We recruited those patients who were interested in using the app and provided each of them with a unique code that enabled activation of the app free of charge when downloaded from the NHS App Library. The only exclusion criterion included the inability to understand English. Control group data was collected for a previous study assessing group educational sessions,

---

[10] Lyzwinski LN. A systematic review and meta-analysis of mobile devices and weight loss with an intervention content analysis. J Pers Med 2014 Jun 30;4(3):311-385 [FREE Full text] [CrossRef] [Medline]

with the participants attending the service between 2016 and 2019. The duration of follow-up for the control group was 6 months.

Each recruited participant had ongoing clinical input and follow-up with members of our hospital-based (tier 3) obesity management team as part of usual care throughout the study period. Although conceived and commenced within the pre–COVID-19 era (January 2020), there was substantial overlap of much of our study with the COVID-19 pandemic (for five of the seven months of the study period, between March and September 2020). As a result, no patient in the tier 3 weight management service received specialist dietary input from March 2020 onward. The clinical follow-up varied between patients, but most received telephone review by a doctor 6 months after the previous appointment. However, the Low Carb Program app supported each participant with invitations to virtual meetups every Monday to provide an opportunity for social connection with other users during the "lockdown" period in the United Kingdom. We conducted the virtual meetups through coach-led video conferencing sessions that provided an informal space for the sharing of personal experiences and establishment of peer support networks.

How Does Personalization Appear?

For the purposes of our study, we used a streamlined version of the Low Carb Program app, specifically personalized to people living with obesity within the community. An example of personalization is shown here:

> Patient A is a 60-year-old South Asian female diagnosed with morbid obesity and comorbidities. Patient A speaks Hindi as her first language and is a vegetarian. On signing up to the program, Patient A's registration data personalizes her experience of the app. Patient A is presented with structured education that explains the physiology of obesity

and comorbidities and how to self-manage a healthy weight. Patient A's experience is provided in Hindi, delivering information to meet cultural needs and expectations. Patient A is supported with vegetarian meal plans that are provided in Punjabi and ingredients that match cultural expectations. Virtual meetups that Patient A engages in are facilitated by a Hindi-speaking coach should she choose to engage with this component of the app.

Patient B is a 52-year-old Caucasian male diagnosed with obesity and prediabetes. Patient B speaks English as his first language, is a smoker, eats a standard diet, and is allergic to dairy. On signing up to the program, Patient B's registration data personalizes his experience of the app. Patient B is presented with structured education that explains the physiology of prediabetes and how to self-manage prediabetes. Patient B's experience is provided in English. Patient B is supported with meal plans that exclude dairy and are provided in English. Virtual meetups that Patient B engages in are facilitated by an English-speaking coach should he choose to engage with this component of the app.

Results

Participants exhibited a mean baseline body weight of 130.2 (SD 29.2) kg, a mean age of 48.8 (SD 12.7) years, and a mean HbA1c of 48.0 (SD 15.5) mmol/mol. The majority of participants (n=62, 59 percent) were female. A minority of participants (n=38, 36.9 percent) had diabetes mellitus (type 1 diabetes: n=5; T2D: n=33). The baseline phenotype of app users was broadly similar to the retrospective control group in terms of baseline weight, proportion of patients with diabetes, and baseline HbA1c, but was significantly different in terms of age and gender.

Of the recruited participants (n=105), all enrolled in the Low Carb Program app. Overall, 90 of the 105 participants (86 percent) completed the Low Carb Program app registration process and engaged with the Low Carb Program app program. A total of 88 participants (84 percent) actively engaged with the Low Carb Program app within the previous 30 days. Only a minority of participants (19/105, 18 percent) completed the entire Low Carb Program app program (defined as completing 9 or more of the 12 education modules available). A total of 58 of the 105 recruited participants (55 percent) self-reported outcomes from the Low Carb Program app. Of the 47 participants who did not self-report outcomes, 29 participants (62 percent) were actively using the Low Carb Program app at follow-up assessments. The mean duration between baseline (registration) and follow-up check-in to self-report HbA1c and body weight was 5 months. Half of all participants engaged with the Low Carb Program app between 3 and 7 months (range 1–12 months). The mean duration of clinical follow-up for recruited participants who received the Low Carb Program app was 7.4 months.

Paired data was available from 48 Low Carb Program app users for body weight and 41 Low Carb Program app users for HbA1c. Paired sample test analysis revealed a statistically significant mean loss of body weight of 2.7 kg (P=.001) and improvement in HbA1c of 3.3 mmol/mol (P=.01). The mean percentage weight loss of the whole cohort was 2.5 percent, with 10 of 48 patients (20.8 percent of our sample) achieving weight loss of more than 5 percent and 18 of 48 patients (23 percent of our sample) achieving weight loss of at least 3 percent.

Data comparisons between the Low Carb Program app user group and the pre–COVID-19 retrospective control group (usual clinical care) revealed similar loss of body weight and change in HbA1c between the two groups. The mean percentage weight loss in the control group was 0.88

percent, with 15 of 92 (16.3 percent) patients achieving weight loss of more than 5 percent. This is in keeping with the statistical test that showed that there was no statistically significant difference in the weight loss between the app group and the retrospective group.

Discussion

Our data confirms equivalence of body weight reduction resulting from remote obesity management complemented by digitally enabled support through the Low Carb Program app versus traditional face-to-face hospital-based obesity management implemented during the pre–COVID-19 era. This is a novel insight that has important implications for the future delivery and hybridized digitalization of hospital-based obesity services. Our data corroborates a recent meta-analysis on mobile app interventions, showing similar reductions in body weight and improvements in glycemic control.[11] The clinical relevance of this study is the impact of digital tools on weight loss and the need to incorporate them into the NHS obesity pathways. Meaningful improvements in blood glucose levels and dyslipidemia are seen with a weight loss of 3 percent or more.[12, 13] In our cohort, 23 percent (18/48) had a weight loss of more than 3 percent, and this will translate into meaningful clinical improvements

---

[11] Wang Y, Min J, Khuri J, Xue H, Xie B, A Kaminsky L, et al. Effectiveness of Mobile Health Interventions on Diabetes and Obesity Treatment and Management: Systematic Review of Systematic Reviews. JMIR mHealth uHealth 2020 Apr 28;8(4):e15400.

[12] Diabetes Prevention Program Research Group, Knowler WC, Fowler SE, Hamman RF, Christophi CA, Hoffman HJ, et al. 10-year follow-up of diabetes incidence and weight loss in the Diabetes Prevention Program Outcomes Study. Lancet 2009 Nov 14;374(9702):1677–1686.

[13] Wing RR, Lang W, Wadden TA, Safford M, Knowler WC, Bertoni AG, et al. Benefits of modest weight loss in improving cardiovascular risk factors in overweight and obese individuals with type 2 diabetes. Diabetes Care 2011 Jul;34(7):1481–1486.

in blood glucose, as well as improvements in dyslipidemia. Moreover, we should not underestimate the utility of any weight loss on the emotional and psychological status of people who struggle with their weight. This can have great motivational effects, and the fact that this was "self-induced," without any active input from a dietitian, means it is likely to also improve self-esteem and self-confidence, which in turn should help to encourage further weight loss over time.

It is important to highlight the serendipitous nature of our study, with its conception and initiation prior to the emergence of COVID-19 onto the world stage. Although originally designed as a means to complement the traditional standard of face-to-face, multidisciplinary management of obesity delivered within a hospital-based setting, use of the Low Carb Program app instead complemented the remote delivery of obesity management delivered over the telephone by a diminished team (without focused dietetic support), due to the obstructive effects of the COVID-19 pandemic. Thus, the execution of our study morphed out of a necessity to adapt and align our clinical practice in response to a global pandemic, in combination with a study design in which COVID-19 did not feature. In retrospect, the Low Carb Program app seems more apt to complement a remote care model than one of a traditional (pre–COVID-19) standard of care. Furthermore, during the COVID-19 pandemic, none of our patients received any dietetic support due to staff redeployment at UHCW. Therefore, we cannot attribute the changes in body weight and HbA1c observed with the Low Carb Program app and remote management to any dietetic input. Conversely, these clinical outcomes stemmed from remote medical and psychological input combined with patient engagement with the Low Carb Program app (including learned education, knowledge, and lifestyle behavioral and dietary changes).

The Low Carb Program app had a high sign-up rate, with all participants signing up (105/105, 100 percent), and a high engagement rate at follow-up (88/105, 83.8 percent). Overall, 15 of the 105 participants (14.3 percent) did not complete the registration process, and 47 of the

105 participants (44.8 percent) did not report outcomes once they had activated their registration. However, much of this group (29/47, 61.7 percent) were actively using the app at follow-up. These results suggest that the intervention requires adaptations to fully engage patients diagnosed with obesity and that other features of the app may be more engaging than health tracking.

Our study had several limitations. Because of the observational nature of our study and its design as a clinical innovation, there was no randomization and no inclusion of a control (placebo) group for direct comparison with those participants who engaged with the Low Carb Program app in combination with remotely delivered obesity management. Although it is possible that the clinical benefits of this combination stemmed solely from the remote interactions with members of the obesity team, this seems unlikely given the notable absence of any focused support from specialist dieticians. A much more likely scenario is that engagement with the Low Carb Program app helped to complement remote management in patients' achievements of clinical outcomes. Furthermore, although we did not include a control group, we did make comparisons retrospectively with a group of patients who had received a traditional standard of care pre–COVID-19. As this study assessed the feasibility of the app, we did not collect information on medication changes that future studies should capture. Change in glycemic therapy could be a confounder, given the effects of SGLT2 inhibitors and GLP1 analogs on body weight. Additionally, data on BMI was not available for all participants, and therefore we did not include it as part of this pilot study.

Conclusion

Our evaluation provides the first proof of concept for digitalized specialist obesity management within a hospital-based (tier 3) obesity service. We demonstrate the clinical efficacy of such an approach, both regarding loss of body weight and improvement in glycemic control. Future studies should explore how to adapt the app to populations seen within the clinical obesity setting to improve user engagement and long-term outcomes. Ultimately, the app represents a management option that is potentially both accessible and scalable at the population level. From a preventive perspective, the Low Carb Program app has relevance for the general population, regardless of obesity status.

A healthy lifestyle is important for all of us. After all, an ounce of prevention is worth a pound of cure.

Building on Our Evidence

Because of the success of the initial partnership between the hospital obesity service and digital therapeutic provider, the wider team came together to co-develop W8Buddy, the first digital support tool developed specifically for NHS Tier 3 Weight Management Services.

W8Buddy provides a precision tier 3 weight management service (T3WMS) to support patients to achieve their self-selected health goals and clinically meaningful weight loss with real-time remote monitoring capabilities.

The service was developed by the entire specialist weight management (obesity) multidisciplinary team at University Hospital Coventry and Warwickshire (weight management dietitians, psychologists, and physicians led by Dr. Petra Hanson, NIHR clinical lecturer in diabetes and endocrinology, MBChB, BSc, MRCP, FHEA, PhD), feedback from people within the NHS obesity clinical service, and DDM Health, providers of NHS-trusted digital technologies.

The platform provides features including structured education, coaching, community, health and goal tracking, meal and food logging (including taking photos of food), recipes, on-demand activity classes tailored to fitness level, and real-time remote home monitoring.

The Gro Health intervention is available on the Web (responsive), smartphone app (iOS/Android), and smart assistants/TVs with an offline pack supporting digitally excluded users.

Visually impaired users are supported with full WCAG 2.1 compliance, compatibility with all screen readers/visual app readers, larger/bolder fonts, audio-only content, editing of themes (dark mode) to reduce eye stress, voice-activated Alexa/Google app, and ability to cast/AirPlay the app to their TV. Users with hearing impairments receive subtitled/BSL-signed videos, offline learning materials, and coaching with interpreters.

The platform has been deployed across the T3WMS.

Further still, the platform is being utilized in other areas of care within the hospital including cardiac rehabilitation, cancer care, and type 1 diabetes.

Understanding People's Attitudes Toward Data for the Optimization of a Specialist Podiatry Service for People with Long-Term Health Conditions

The following case study presents a best-practice example of how to listen to an audience at scale to understand attitudes, preferences, and digital personas concerning an intended technology and its ramifications.

More than 77,000 diabetics in England have foot ulcers today.[14] The longer ulcers progress, the longer they take to heal. If untreated, ulcers can lead to diabetic foot disease (DFD) and amputation. Twenty-five people in England have a lower limb (toe/foot/leg) amputated daily; tragically, 85 percent of these are preventable. From 2015–2018, 27,465 lower limb

---

[14] GOV.UK. (n.d.). National diabetic foot care report. [online] Available at: https://www.gov.uk/government/statistics/national-diabetic-foot-care-report.

diabetes-related amputations happened in England (up 18.3 percent from 2011–2014), and 147,067 hospital admissions for DFD were recorded with an average 8-day stay totaling 1,826,734 hospital bed days at the cost of £376/day.[15]

The foot check is a chance for potential problems to be identified and assessed and preventive action taken. NICE NG19 states people with diabetes should have annual foot checks and recommends patients with active foot problems be referred to a multidisciplinary team/foot protection service within one working day and triaged within another working day.[16] Yet there is "poor symptom recognition by the patient, inaccurate health care assessment, and difficulties in accessing specialist services" due to the following:

- *Delays to exam*: The National Diabetes Foot Audit found 39 percent of people waited 14+ days for their first foot ulceration specialist examination.

- *Lack of testing*: 800,000 patients in England do not get an annual foot check, and 80 percent of practice nurses who conduct foot checks need to be more confident in performing them, causing variances in care and outcomes.

- *Training*: 33 percent of NHS commissioners in England do not provide HCPs with footcare training, and where training is in place, the quality of the assessment could be better.

---

[15] The Diabetes Times. (2020). Diabetes-related lower limb amputations up by 18%. [online] Available at: https://diabetestimes.co.uk/diabetes-related-lower-limb-amputations-up-by-18-per-cent/.

[16] NICE (2015). Overview | Diabetic foot problems: prevention and management | Guidance | NICE. [online] Nice.org.uk. Available at: https://www.nice.org.uk/guidance/ng19.

There is a drastic need for support to reduce the clinical and economic impact of DFD and a massive opportunity for digital health innovation to democratize care and outcomes through the following:

- Reducing time to examination and thus untreated ulceration/DFD

- Conducting/supporting the foot check itself to support clinical decision-making

- Providing training/education, resources, and treatment for healthcare professionals and patients between annual checks

There is a significant economic benefit to be realized, too: a 30 percent bed-days reduction from reduced ulceration would save the NHS £63.5m/year. That was before the COVID-19 pandemic, which saw an increase in urgent foot health problems and a decline in face-to-face patient volume and impacted clinicians' mental health. Smartphones provide a vital opportunity to extend care. However, there are very few apps supporting ulceration and foot care.

As well as the technologies themselves, the data they generate is helpful. While the exceptional measures implemented in some countries to combat coronavirus may prove effective in limiting the spread of the virus, some provoked controversy in terms of privacy and other fundamental rights with respect to data, particularly when they lack transparency and public consultation. Surprisingly, evidence on sharing clinical trial or public health research data is limited while remaining a stalwart of many digital systems.

FootChecker is a multiplatform app for healthcare professionals and patients to reduce foot ulceration, amputations, recovery time, and associated costs by standardizing clinician confidence and ability and providing risk-stratified patient education for assessment, advice, and early intervention to patients.

Objective

Our study aimed to understand the opinions of British people with long-term health conditions on the themes of data privacy and security, data ethics, and data misuse. It is essential to understand the concerns of people with long-term health conditions such as type 2 diabetes and hypertension, as these conditions are key risk factors in the progression and prognosis of ulceration. This was confounded during the pandemic, as both type 2 diabetes and hypertension are also COVID-19 morbidity and mortality risk factors.

Methods

A web-based survey study was conducted with a mixed-methods design conforming to the checklist for reporting results of electronic Internet surveys. People 18 and older who had joined the Diabetes.co.uk community were surveyed. An email invitation to participate, which included a web link to the study, was sent to 11,213 people who had consented to be contacted for research opportunities.

The survey commenced with one screening question: "Do you consent to participate in the study?" Respondents who consented went on to complete the survey. Quantitative information (closed and multiple-choice questions) was collected on demographic characteristics, clinical diagnoses, and sharing and privacy of pre– and post–COVID-19 health data. We conducted descriptive data analyses of sample distributions and characteristics. Pearson r correlation coefficients were used to determine the relationship between prior data-sharing behavior and attitudes toward data-sharing activity in the context of the COVID-19 pandemic. The data from the open question was read and then categorized into themes.

Results

Of 11,213 people who emailed, 10,705 clicked through to the survey; in total, 4,764 gave their consent and began the study. All respondents completed the survey and were included in the analysis. All respondents were located in the United Kingdom. In total, 2,287 (48.0 percent) respondents were male, and 3,083 (64.8 percent) were aged between 55 and 74. 115 (2.8 percent) respondents reported having been clinically diagnosed with COVID-19. Most patients (n=4674, 98.1 percent) reported a prior clinical diagnosis of at least one health condition (on average, three per person). There was a high prevalence of individuals living with type 2 diabetes (n=2974, 62.7 percent), hypertension (n=2147, 45.2 percent), type 1 diabetes (n=1299, 27.4), obesity (n=892, 18.8 percent), and depression (n=871, 18.3 percent).

Before the COVID-19 pandemic, almost half of the respondents (n=2313, 49.2 percent) agreed or strongly agreed that they often consented to the anonymized sharing of their private health data. In comparison, only 608 (13 percent) respondents often consented to sharing private health data without anonymization. Two-thirds of respondents (n=3113, 66.7 percent) disagreed or strongly disagreed with sharing their personal health data without anonymization. Similarly, 3,121 (66.3 percent) respondents would share their data if it keeps other people healthy; 3,026 (63.9 percent) respondents agreed or strongly agreed to share private health data with the government or health authority; 1,911 (40.7 percent) respondents agreed or strongly agreed to share their private health data with services that provide health services to the National Health Service (NHS) such as the Low Carb Program and PushDoctor. Only 232 (5 percent) participants agreed or strongly agreed to share private health data with social media platforms.

More than a quarter of respondents (n=1297, 27.8 percent) agreed or strongly agreed that they did not trust any organization to protect their private health data. Just under a quarter of respondents (n=1094, 23.5

percent) agreed or strongly agreed that they were not concerned by the implications of sharing private health data. Respondents who reported feeling "neutral" in response to the statements were excluded.

More than half (n=3026, 63.9 percent) agreed or strongly agreed to share their private data with the government or health authority if asked; 1,911 (40.7 percent) respondents would happily consent to share their private data with services that provide health services to the NHS such as the Low Carb Program and if asked. Only 232 (5 percent) participants agreed or strongly agreed that they would consent to share private data with social media if requested.

Almost half of the respondents (n=2228, 47.1 percent) were concerned or very concerned about who would have access to their health data in the context of the COVID-19 pandemic, and 2,310 (49.1 percent) respondents were concerned or very concerned about how their personal health data may be used in the future. Almost two-thirds of respondents (n=3054, 65 percent) were concerned or very concerned about the legislation regarding data misuse.

Just over a third of respondents (n=1563, 33.4 percent) would consent to share their private data with any organization if it provided essential COVID-19 support services, such as supermarkets, pharmacies, and banks.

Discussion

Our study provides insights into public perception and attitudes toward the use of identifiable health data in the context of the COVID-19 pandemic, in particular, the perspectives of those living with chronic, long-term health conditions, with an average of four health conditions reported per respondent.

Our study suggests that data sensitivity is highly contextual. Many people felt that their attitudes have shifted due to the COVID-19 pandemic. More people reported being comfortable with sharing private health data with any organization rather than before the COVID-19 pandemic. People appear to trust their data with the government and health organizations. There is significant distrust of private health data use by social media organizations (e.g., Twitter, Facebook, and Google) even though social media is used as a channel for communication by people caught up in crises such as emergency relief operations after earthquakes, tsunamis, and typhoons, where it provides a trusted and highly salient source of information about what is happening and what to do.[17, 18]

This is surprising as although users worldwide report that privacy and use of personal data are important issues, most rarely make an effort actively to protect this data and often even give it away voluntarily on social media, where even innocuous data can reveal sensitive health information when suitably processed.[19, 20] People treat data revelation and sharing differently depending on the perceived sensitivity of the data, and the sensitivity attached to different data types is neither stable nor uniform.

[17] Palen L, Hughes AL. Social Media in Disaster Communication. In: Handbook of Disaster Research. Cham: Springer; 2017:497–518.

[18] Muniz-Rodriguez K, Ofori SK, Bayliss LC, Schwind JS, Diallo K, Liu M, et al. Social Media Use in Emergency Response to Natural Disasters: A Systematic Review With a Public Health Perspective. Disaster Med Public Health Prep 2020 Feb 09;14(1):139–149.

[19] Gerber N, Gerber P, Volkamer M. Explaining the privacy paradox: A systematic review of literature investigating privacy attitude and behavior. Comput Secur 2018 Aug;77:226–261.

[20] Raij A, Ghosh A, Kumar S, Srivastava M. Privacy risks emerging from the adoption of innocuous wearable sensors in the mobile environment. 2011 Presented at: CHI '11: CHI Conference on Human Factors in Computing Systems; May 7–12, 2011; Vancouver, BC.

A key theme emerging from the literature confirmed in this study is the importance of trust.[21, 22, 23] More than a quarter of respondents stated they did not trust any organization to protect their data, more than half reported concern about the implications of sharing personal information, and almost two-thirds were concerned about data misuse regulation not being strict enough. When asked during the pandemic (the United Kingdom's first wave), nearly half of respondents were concerned about who would have access to their personal health data, and a similar number were concerned about how their personal health data might be used in the future. This is consistent with prior research suggesting that public involvement in data policy is crucial to bolstering trust and provides support for legislation that is more enforceable.[24] Attitudes may have been perturbed by news stories about cybersecurity and privacy and by policy announcements (e.g., around Huawei, the Online Harms Bill, etc.).[25, 26]

---

[21] Bargain O, Aminjonov U. Trust and compliance to public health policies in times of COVID-19. J Public Econ 2020 Dec;192:104316

[22] Ienca M, Vayena E. On the responsible use of digital data to tackle the COVID-19 pandemic. Nat Med 2020 Apr 27;26(4):463–464

[23] Bunker D. Who do you trust? The digital destruction of shared situational awareness and the COVID-19 infodemic. Int J Inf Manage 2020 Dec;55:102201

[24] Liabo K, Boddy K, Bortoli S, Irvine J, Boult H, Fredlund M, et al. Public involvement in health research: what does 'good' look like in practice? Res Involv Engagem 2020 Mar 31;6(1):11

[25] Lysne O. Containment of Untrusted Modules. In: The Huawei and Snowden Questions. Cham: Springer; 2018:99–107.

[26] Consultation outcome: Online Harms White Paper. Department for Digital, Culture, Media & Sport. Government of the United Kingdom. 2020 Dec 15. https://www.gov.uk/government/consultations/online-harms-white-paper/online-harms-white-paper [accessed 2022-06-01]

Although there are no directly comparable studies, the results from this study complement prior research on public perceptions about COVID-19 and data sharing. Data privacy and protection are essential concepts.[27] Data policy tends to address human concerns about privacy by making rules about data protection; however, this can lead to category errors since data protection can undermine privacy.

Willingness to share anonymized personal health information varies depending on the degree to which the receiving body is trusted and the uses to which the data will be put.[28, 29] The more commercial the objectives of the receiving institution appear, the fewer respondents are willing to share their personal health information. This suggests that anonymization's disadvantages (in terms of confirming data and correlating shared with other data) might be offset by better (broader, deeper, and more accurate) sampling, leading to greater validity of results. Further evidence comes from the interaction (or correlation) between these attitudinal responses and other characteristics, meaning that nonanonymized collection might lead to biased results.

Conclusion

Data sensitivity is highly contextual. More people are comfortable with sharing anonymized data than personally identifiable data. Willingness to share data also varied depending on the receiving body, highlighting trust

---

[27] Zwitter A, Gstrein OJ. Big data, privacy and COVID-19 – learning from humanitarian expertise in data protection. Int J Humanitarian Action 2020 May 18;5(1).

[28] Ghafur S, Van Dael J, Leis M, Darzi A, Sheikh A. Public perceptions on data sharing: key insights from the UK and the USA. Lancet Digit Health 2020 Sep;2(9):e444-e446.

[29] Panesar A. Machine Learning and AI Ethics. In: Machine Learning and AI for Healthcare: Big Data for Improved Health Outcomes. Berkeley, CA: Apress; Dec 16, 2020:207–247.

as a critical theme, who may have access to shared personal health data, and how it may be used in the future. The nascency of legal guidance in this area suggests the requirement for humanitarian guidelines for data responsibility during disaster relief operations such as pandemics and the necessity to involve the public in their development.

Impact of the Findings

The survey findings provided a stark view of public attitudes toward data sharing. Consequentially, to develop and maintain trust, credibility, and engagement, ultimately the development team made several enhancements to the digital tool, including the following:

- Using an "as much data as required" approach to data collected so as not to dissuade users from engaging with the tool

- Providing "simple" terms and conditions to users to ensure all data-sharing aspects are understood

- Providing a mechanism for users to delete all of their data from within the digital app, separate from deleting their user profile

- Providing reinforcement messaging at critical points along the foot-checking journey to re-iterate to whom data is visible, for how long, and which data is made visible

- In-depth information on the security and privacy of all information

Subsequently, the digital platform saw an increase in the number of participants completing the registration process by 213 percent.

Evaluation of a Digital Intervention for the Self-Management of Type 2 Diabetes and Prediabetes

The following case study presents the impact of a primary care–delivered precision health tool.

Type 2 diabetes is a costly, chronic, noncommunicable disease expected to affect 552 million people globally by 2030.[30] Globally, the burden of type 2 diabetes is estimated to exceed US $1.3 trillion.[31] In the developed world, individuals living with diabetes are managed by primary care teams, with medical consultation visits averaging less than 3 hours a year. Individuals are essentially on their own most of the time.[32] Because of this enormous gap between appointments, diabetes care is primarily dependent on personal self-management, which, if not performed, increases the risk of premature death, blindness, amputation, and kidney failure.[33] In reality, type 2 diabetes self-management is neither easy nor straightforward and requires time, numeracy, and literacy skills.[34]

---

[30] Whiting DR, Guariguata L, Weil C, Shaw J. IDF diabetes atlas: Global estimates of the prevalence of diabetes for 2011 and 2030. Diabetes Res Clin Pract 2011 Dec;94(3):311-321

[31] Bommer C, Heesemann E, Sagalova V, Manne-Goehler J, Atun R, Bärnighausen T, et al. The global economic burden of diabetes in adults aged 20-79 years: A cost-of-illness study. Lancet Diabetes Endocrinol 2017 Jun;5(6):423–430

[32] Roberts S. Working Together for Better Diabetes Care: Clinical Case for Change. Report. London, UK: Department of Health; 2007.

[33] Harris MI. Health care and health status and outcomes for patients with type 2 diabetes. Diabetes Care 2000 Jun;23(6):754–758

[34] Osborn CY, Cavanaugh K, Wallston KA, Rothman RL. Self-efficacy links health literacy and numeracy to glycemic control. J Health Commun 2010;15 Suppl 2:146-158

As with many noncommunicable diseases, lifestyle is one of the leading causes of prediabetes and type 2 diabetes, and improvements in parameters such as dietary composition, physical activity, and sedentary lifestyle are determinants for reducing the frequency of this type of pathology.

Losing weight can provide significant health benefits, and losing excess body weight reduces the risk of type 2 diabetes, heart disease, osteoarthritis, and sleep apnea.[35] In addition, the maintenance of reasonable blood glucose control has benefits for patients, with every 1 percent (6.2 mmol/mol) reduction in hemoglobin A1c (HbA1c) contributing to a 43 percent reduction in the risk of amputation, 14 percent reduction in risk of myocardial infarction, and 37 percent reduction in risk of microvascular complications.[36]

A recent systematic review and meta-analysis of published and unpublished randomized trial data evaluating low-carbohydrate diets (<130 g/day or <26 percent of a 2000 kcal/day diet) and very low–carbohydrate diets (<10 percent calories from carbohydrates) for at least 12 weeks in adults with type 2 diabetes found that based on moderate- to low-certainty evidence, patients adhering to a low-carbohydrate diet for six months may experience remission of type 2 diabetes without adverse consequences.[37]

---

[35] National Institute of Diabetes and Digestive and Kidney Diseases. 2018. https://www.niddk.nih.gov/health-information/weight-management/adult-overweight-obesity/health-risks [accessed 2021-08-10]

[36] Stratton IM, Adler AI, Neil HA, Matthews DR, Manley SE, Cull CA, et al. Association of glycaemia with macrovascular and microvascular complications of type 2 diabetes (UKPDS 35): Prospective observational study. BMJ 2000 Aug 12;321(7258):405–412

[37] Goldenberg JZ, Day A, Brinkworth GD, Sato J, Yamada S, Jönsson T, et al. Efficacy and safety of low and very low carbohydrate diets for type 2 diabetes remission: Systematic review and meta-analysis of published and unpublished randomized trial data. BMJ 2021 Jan 13;372:m4743

Integrating digital technology into primary care can increase access to care, improve patient outcomes, and decrease costs. Digital technology, including smartphone apps, can potentially augment and extend the reach of health services through self-management support impacting lifestyle behaviors.[38] Smartphone apps have been demonstrated to improve glycemic outcomes in people with type 1 and type 2 diabetes.[39] Although there is evidence to the contrary, of the 23 studies analyzed in the systematic review published by Schoeppe et al. on the efficacy of apps in improving lifestyle, smartphones were seen to have a favorable impact on food habits in only five studies. They resulted in increased physical activity in nine studies.[40] Even though recent systematic reviews have concluded that Internet and mobile interventions can improve lifestyle behaviors, most studies had at most 3 to 6 months of follow-up, which emphasizes the need for research in long-term interventions.[41]

---

[38] Hoffman L, Benedetto E, Huang H, Grossman E, Kaluma D, Mann Z, et al. Augmenting mental health in primary care: A 1-year study of deploying smartphone apps in a multi-site primary care/behavioral health integration program. Front Psychiatry 2019;10:94

[39] Offringa R, Sheng T, Parks L, Clements M, Kerr D, Greenfield MS. Digital diabetes management application improves glycemic outcomes in people with type 1 and type 2 diabetes. J Diabetes Sci Technol 2018 May;12(3):701–708

[40] Schoeppe S, Alley S, Van Lippevelde W, Bray NA, Williams SL, Duncan MJ, et al. Efficacy of interventions that use apps to improve diet, physical activity and sedentary behaviour: A systematic review. Int J Behav Nutr Phys Act 2016 Dec 07;13(1):127

[41] Romeo A, Edney S, Plotnikoff R, Curtis R, Ryan J, Sanders I, et al. Can smartphone apps increase physical activity? Systematic review and meta-analysis. J Med Internet Res 2019 Mar 19;21(3):e12053

Interventions providing low-carbohydrate or very low–carbohydrate programs have been clinically demonstrated to support improvements in weight, blood glucose, and demedication.[42, 43] Further still, the diets are associated with improvements in acute and chronic pain, depression, anxiety, and stress.[44, 45, 46]

Long-term studies of low-carbohydrate dietary approaches to treat type 2 diabetes and obesity are limited, particularly those delivered and supported remotely.[47]

Objectives

With therapeutic carbohydrate restriction demonstrating significant benefits in improving symptoms of chronic disease, this real-world study was conducted to evaluate the effectiveness of a digitally delivered digital

---

[42] Bolla, Caretto, Laurenzi, Scavini, Piemonti. Low-carb and ketogenic diets in type 1 and type 2 diabetes. Nutrients 2019 Apr 26;11(5):962

[43] Sato J, Kanazawa A, Makita S, Hatae C, Komiya K, Shimizu T, et al. A randomized controlled trial of 130 g/day low-carbohydrate diet in type 2 diabetes with poor glycemic control. Clin Nutr 2017 Aug;36(4):992–1000.

[44] Nielsen JV, Joensson E. Low-carbohydrate diet in type 2 diabetes. Stable improvement of bodyweight and glycemic control during 22 months follow-up. Nutr Metab (Lond) 2006 Jun 14;3:22

[45] Athinarayanan SJ, Adams RN, Hallberg S, Phinney S, McKenzie A. Effect of a continuous remote care intervention on glycemic target achievement and medication use among adults with T2D: A post hoc analysis. In: Proceedings of the American Diabetes Association (ADA) 80th Scientific Sessions. 2020 Jun Presented at: American Diabetes Association (ADA) 80th Scientific Sessions; June 12–16, 2020; Virtual.

[46] Saslow LR, Summers C, Aikens JE, Unwin DJ. Outcomes of a digitally delivered low-carbohydrate type 2 diabetes self-management program: 1-year results of a single-arm longitudinal study. JMIR Diabetes 2018 Aug 03;3(3):e12

[47] Torous, J., Lipschitz, J., Ng, M. and Firth, J., 2020. Dropout rates in clinical trials of smartphone apps for depressive symptoms: a systematic review and meta-analysis. Journal of affective disorders, 263, pp.413–419.

therapeutic intervention at 12 months on the maintenance of glycemic control for NHS-recruited patients at Norwood Surgery in Southport, United Kingdom.

Methods

We used a single-arm pre-post-intervention study design. Participants were not paid for participation and were given access to the program for free. Participants provided informed consent regarding their anonymized data being used for analysis and publication.

Participants were recruited from an NHS primary care setting—Norwood Surgery in Southport, United Kingdom—between April 19, 2018, and August 19, 2019. Patients aged 18 years or older with a confirmed diagnosis of type 2 diabetes or prediabetes who presented for any reason during the recruitment window were eligible for signposting if the consulting healthcare professional felt appropriate.

Patients who accepted signposting were given a Low Carb Program referral card, which patients redeemed on the app or website. To have broad applicability to a nonclinical trial setting, the only de facto exclusion criterion was the inability to understand English. One hundred referral cards were provided to the NHS general practice in Southport. A total of 45 participants signed up, and all were followed for 12 months. The characteristics of the 55 participants who declined the referral card were not recorded.

For a baseline, participants recruited to the Low Carb Program input their type of diabetes, year of diagnosis, most recent HbA1c test result and date, age, gender, socioeconomic status based on household income, and presence of comorbid chronic illnesses at sign-up. At 12 months, participants were again asked to report on their current HbA1c level and weight.

Results

Of the 45 baseline participants who activated their referral, 37 (82 percent) reported outcomes at 12 months. For the remaining eight people (18 percent) lost to follow-up, the last recorded data point was carried forward to maintain a conservative real-world evaluation.

Participants with type 2 diabetes who were recruited to the Low Carb Program showed a statistically significant change in HbA1c from baseline (mean 73.35 mmol/mol, SD 15.84) to 12-month follow-up (mean 67.2 mmol/mol, SD 13.59), equivalent to a mean reduction of 6.2 mmol/mol (SD 5.75; t17=4.56; P<.001). Participants who completed more than nine lessons of the program showed a statistically significant decrease in HbA1c from baseline (mean 75.7 mmol/mol, SD 14.9) to 12-month follow-up (mean 68.7 mmol/mol, SD 12.8), a mean reduction in HbA1c of 7.01 mmol/mol (SD 6.06; t13=4.33; P<.001). This is equivalent to an 8.81 percent mean reduction in HbA1c. Participants with prediabetes who were recruited to the Low Carb Program showed a statistically significant mean reduction in HbA1c of 2.35 mmol/mol (SD 1.96; t26=6.25; P<.001). Those participants who completed more than nine of the lessons did even better, reporting a mean HbA1c reduction of 3.04 mmol/mol (SD 1.82) at 12 months (t17=7.11; P<.001)

Participants with type 2 diabetes had an average starting weight of 93.53 kg (SD 17.91) that dropped to an average of 90.83 kg (SD 16.84) at the 12-month follow-up, which is a statistically significant mean reduction of 2.70 kg (SD 2.21; t17=5.17; P<.001). Completers reduced their weight by an average of 3.54 kg (SD 1.7; t17=5.17; P<.001), equivalent to a mean body weight change of –3.66 percent (SD 2.8). Participants with prediabetes started the program with a mean weight of 86.72 kg (SD 9.68) and reported an average weight loss of 2.82 kg (SD 2.90; t26=5.05; P<.001), equivalent to a mean body weight decrease of 3.16 percent (SD 3.11). Participants with prediabetes who completed more than nine lessons of the program demonstrated a greater statistically significant change in mean body weight of 4.08 kg (SD 2.77; t17=6.25; P<.001), equivalent to a mean reduction in overall body weight of 4.57 percent (SD 2.88).

149

Discussion

This was not a randomized controlled trial, so we cannot compare the 12-month results to a control or standard-of-care group. Therefore, the results of our trial should be interpreted cautiously because this small study used convenience sampling, an open-label single-arm design, and pre-post self-reported outcomes. However, this study demonstrated that signposting patients with type 2 diabetes or prediabetes to the Low Carb Program as part of routine general practice care can promote weight loss and improve glycemic control. With minimal implementation and support, this light-touch intervention was able to augment primary care workflows. It demonstrated high uptake, adherence (i.e., completion), and retention (i.e., engagement within the last 30 days) of 45 percent, 64 percent, and 82 percent, respectively. There was a low dropout rate (8/45, 18 percent) at 12 months, demonstrating high platform engagement. It is one of the few apps to show long-term engagement. The platform has been shown to have a high engagement rate and to be noninferior to other in-person or online interventions.[48, 49, 50] Given the brief intervention provided, we achieved high uptake within the context of general practice and primary care. Typically, other interventions require staff resources and time.

[48] Griauzde D, Kullgren JT, Liestenfeltz B, Ansari T, Johnson EH, Fedewa A, et al. A mobile phone-based program to promote healthy behaviors among adults with prediabetes who declined participation in free diabetes prevention programs: Mixed-methods pilot randomized controlled trial. JMIR Mhealth Uhealth 2019 Jan 09;7(1):e11267

[49] Kelly T, Unwin D, Finucane F. Low-carbohydrate diets in the management of obesity and type 2 diabetes: A review from clinicians using the approach in practice. Int J Environ Res Public Health 2020 Apr 08;17(7):2557

[50] Pamungkas RA, Chamroonsawasdi K. HbA1c reduction and weight-loss outcomes: A systematic review and meta-analysis of community-based intervention trials among patients with type 2 diabetes mellitus. Int J Diabetes Dev Ctries 2019 Jan 7;39(2):394–407.

Conclusion

Although our study design does not support causal conclusions, this real-world evaluation suggests that the intervention can be a valuable adjunct for precision self-management for adults with type 2 diabetes and prediabetes.

Impact of the Findings

An independent health economics report conducted by the York Health Economics Consortium employed real-world data on the impact of the Low Carb Program to demonstrate the significant savings in implementing the Low Carb Program within a public healthcare system. For a local area with 3,000 licenses, researchers modeled that the cost savings at the end of one year of Low Carb Program implementation would save an average of £117.57 per participant in reduced medication. Results have supported the national scaling of the digital multiplatform tool.[51]

Voice-Based Symptom Monitoring and AI-Based Rehabilitation for Patients with Long COVID

The following case study presents an award-winning technical business case for a precision health tool that utilizes AI-based symptom monitoring for monitoring of Long COVID.

---

[51] York Health Economics Consortium. (2021). NHS Innovation Accelerator: Low Carb Program.

151

Background

Long COVID is an illness that has affected 40 percent of the world's 478 million survivors of COVID-19.[52] NICE guidelines recommend directing patients to apps to help with self-management of the condition.[53] The condition is debilitating and can impact mental well-being, family, employment, and quality of life.[54] Healthcare workers have a higher prevalence of Long COVID, with ~2 million days lost in NHS staff absences due to Long COVID annually.[55] Long COVID is the single most significant cause of long-term absence from work.[56] Long COVID affects healthcare workers disproportionately to the general population.[57] Improving rehabilitation times would support people in getting back to work quicker. Employers will benefit from fewer sick days and improved mental health and quality of life. Almost 20 percent of patients will require rehabilitation for 5 to 6 months, with a large volume presenting stress-related problems.

---

[52] Taquet, M., Dercon, Q., Luciano, S., Geddes, J. R., Husain, M., & Harrison, P. J. (2021). Incidence, co-occurrence, and evolution of long-COVID features: A 6-month retrospective cohort study of 273,618 survivors of COVID-19. PLoS medicine, 18(9), e1003773.

[53] Venkatesan, P., 2021. NICE guideline on long COVID. The Lancet Respiratory Medicine, 9(2), p.129.

[54] Davis, H.E., Assaf, G.S., McCorkell, L., Wei, H., Low, R.J., Re'em, Y., Redfield, S., Austin, J.P. and Akrami, A., 2021. Characterizing long COVID in an international cohort: 7 months of symptoms and their impact. EClinicalMedicine, 38, p.101019.

[55] Long Covid: nearly 2m days lost in NHS staff absences in England, The Guardian, 2022. Retrieved from https://www.theguardian.com/society/2022/jan/24/long-covid-nearly-2m-days-lost-in-nhs-staff-absences-in-england.

[56] Strauss, D. (2022). Long Covid now major cause of long-term job absence, say quarter of UK employers. Financial Times. [online] 8 Feb. Available at: https://www.ft.com/content/33444f29-bab1-4655-85b5-c0b1f68d9653.

[57] Nguyen, L. H., Drew, D. A., Graham, M. S., Joshi, A. D., Guo, C. G., Ma, W., ... & Zhang, F. (2020). Risk of COVID-19 among front-line health-care workers and the general community: a prospective cohort study. The Lancet Public Health, 5(9), e475–e483.

Only a handful of rehabilitation apps for long-term conditions are relevant to Long COVID. For example, NHS Wales' Long COVID-specific self-management app provides essential information with little interactivity. Although covering general rehabilitation principles, existing apps lack Long COVID specificity and personalized interactivity. We need ways to reach people equitably to manage Long COVID and support focused rehabilitation and outcomes. Current tools are either informational or a GUI mobile app and do not monitor symptoms or provide support by voice, excluding 60 percent of people over 65, a key Long COVID risk group, who do not use a smartphone.

With AI voice assistants, speech can be transformed into a vital sign, allowing health assessment and symptom-based rehabilitation. In the same way that temperature indicates fever, vocal biomarkers offer a more complete picture of our health.

Automatic sound classification has been widely adopted in various real-life applications, such as health monitoring, security surveillance, environmental sensing, robot navigation, and voice activity. Sound classification tasks involve the extraction of acoustic characteristics from the audio signals and the subsequent identification of different sound classes. The broad range of sound classification deployments can be categorized into several disciplines, including speech recognition, music instrument identification, environmental sound classification, and medical sound classification for disease diagnosis. Compared with speech and music sounds with proper high-level structures, the categories of diagnostic (such as respiratory, coughing, and heart) sounds and environmental audio signals tend to be unstructured, containing various clinical and natural acoustic noises. Furthermore, because of different sound production mechanisms (e.g., different body recording locations and equipment), sound classification with medical audio clips is a challenging problem. It has been rarely tackled in existing literature, particularly concerning lung conditions (e.g., COPD, pneumonia, asthma, and bronchiectasis) and COVID diagnosis using respiratory, coughing, and speech audio signals. Because of highly imbalanced and limited sample sizes, existing studies need better performances. Moreover, owing to the subtlety and notoriously noisy, murky, and fuzzy boundaries of human emotions, emotion recognition from audio inputs is also tricky.

Objective

The objective of our project is to adapt the Gro Health app demonstrated to support a variety of health conditions, meet/exceed equality and diversity aims, and have very high engagement with ethnic minority patient groups, retired adults, and those with learning difficulties. The project will provide personalized rehabilitation exercises based on monitoring Long COVID symptoms through wearable and voice delivered through a chatbot that providers can embed within smart devices, vehicles, and homes.

As the digitalization of health services accelerates, finding routes to connect with the digitally excluded is essential not to exacerbate existing health inequalities. Reducing health inequalities is the core problem our product seeks to solve. The innovation will be available 24/7 on smart devices, including voice assistants and smart TVs, to reach 60 percent of those over 65s without a smartphone, making it the only in-home Long COVID support solution for those without a smartphone.

This project has specific technical challenges, including accuracy of voice capture, potential noises in data analysis, integration of different data points to provide a holistic evaluation of Long COVID, and multidisciplinary self-management support based on autonomic principles.

The developed AI agent will fill a knowledge gap by developing novel weakly supervised, zero-shot (ZSL), and few-shot (FSL) learning and deep learning algorithms to generate effective audio representations to capture significant discriminative spatial-temporal characteristics and acoustic cues to inform audio-based disease and emotion classification.

Machine learning engineers will also employ evolving neural architecture generation techniques to yield bespoke optimized networks to better tackle audio classification with various noisy data inputs.

Implementation Plan

The project is a collaborative relationship between DDM Health and Royal Holloway, University of London, involving the following:

- Collection of data through in-app patient voice and symptom data.

- Mixed-method design consisting of interviews, a voice diary, and data from the Gro Health app with data analysis to capture and analyze how long COVID sufferers' symptoms manifest on physiological and psychological levels.

- Design and develop an interactive AI agent that enables personalized real-time support and self-management recommendations. Core features are monitoring long COVID symptoms by data synchronization with wearable devices, audio recording through the user's manual input, emotion detection from speech, and providing support and coping strategies via an interactive AI agent.

- System evaluation using existing data sets and real-time inputs.

- Report writing and dissemination.

Risks

Technical risks include the following:

- The study team can mitigate insufficient audio data by using many existing respiratory, coughing, and speech public data sets concerning diverse lung abnormalities and COVID detection.

- Slow training processes can be mitigated by using powerful high-performance GPU computing facilities.

- The need for more background knowledge in medical audio classification can be mitigated by drawing significant experiences from the successful delivery of previous projects on system development, conducting a comprehensive literature review, and consulting relevant researchers/NHS partners/domain experts.

Evaluation

University researchers will evaluate the project by working with existing partners to recruit Long COVID patients for a longitudinal mixed-methods evaluation of the AI agent, including health data tracking, questionnaires, and interviews to detail user AI engagement and health impact.

Potential Impact

The impact of the project is far-reaching with potential benefits significant for the following:

- *Patients*: Standardizing access to Long COVID support reduces patient care and outcome variances.

- *Employers*: Long COVID is the single biggest cause of long-term absence from work.[58] Long COVID affects healthcare workers disproportionately to the general population. Improving rehabilitation times would support people in getting back to work quicker. Employers will benefit from fewer sick days, improved mental health, and quality of life.

- *Insurers*: Long COVID is the second most common cause of early intervention and rehabilitation for Group Income Protection policies in 2021.[59] Improving rehabilitation will reduce claims.

Negative impacts include the potential reduction in face-to-face appointments between patients and their healthcare professionals. This will be mitigated through research, including evaluating the burden on healthcare professionals and including relevant stakeholders in developing and delivering the app to ensure user appropriateness.

---

[58] Halpin, S.J., McIvor, C., Whyatt, G., Adams, A., Harvey, O., McLean, L., Walshaw, C., Kemp, S., Corrado, J., Singh, R. and Collins, T., 2021. Postdischarge symptoms and rehabilitation needs in survivors of COVID-19 infection: a cross-sectional evaluation. Journal of medical virology, 93(2), pp.1013–1022.

[59] minutes, 14 A. 2022 2 (2022). Long Covid: now second most supported Aviva Group Income Protection condition. [online] connect.avivab2b.co.uk. Available at: https://connect.avivab2b.co.uk/adviser/articles/news/workplace-and-group-protection/Long-Covid-second-most-supported-condition/.

Developing a Digital Tool to Support Daily Behavioral Change for Children and Young People to Support Healthier Lives

The following case study presents the design and production of a precision health tool to provide child and parent lifestyle and behavioral change health and well-being support. Key aspects of the project involve tackling a societal problem using a data-driven approach, involving all relevant stakeholders in the co-development process, and training staff to deliver the ongoing service.

Being overweight and obese presents significant challenges to our local population's current and future health. Data from the National Child Measurement Programme (NCMP), which involves the weighing and measuring of Reception (age 4–5) and Year 6 (age 10–11) children, highlights that in Cornwall, in 2019/2020, 25.1 percent of Reception and 31.9 percent of Year 6 children were overweight or living with obesity.[60]

Because of the COVID-19 pandemic, in 2020–2021, the NCMP ran a reduced program to collect a nationally representative sample of data. This data showed significant increases in the rates of childhood overweight and obesity nationally (4.7 and 5.7 percentage point increase for Reception and Year 6, respectively); this is the highest annual rise since the NCMP began. If these national increases track into Cornwall, we are approaching one in three children overweight or obese at Reception age. Some groups of

---

[60] NHS (2013). National Child Measurement Programme - NHS Digital. [online] NHS Digital. Available at: https://digital.nhs.uk/services/ national-child-measurement-programme/.

children are disproportionately affected by excess weight. Children living in the most deprived areas are more than twice as likely to be living with obesity than those living in the least deprived areas.[61]

These trends have significant health implications for children in Cornwall. Children who are overweight or obese are at a higher risk of physical health problems, including liver disease, sleep apnea, diabetes, asthma, and orthopedic problems. In addition to physical comorbidities, living with excess weight and obesity is associated with poor psychological and emotional health, with many children experiencing bullying, low self-esteem, body dissatisfaction, and depressive symptoms. Children living with obesity are likely to continue to live with obesity as adults and have a higher risk of morbidity, disability, and premature mortality in adulthood.

Before the COVID-19 pandemic, Healthy Cornwall offered a tier 2 10-week Healthy Families Programme consisting of weekly one-and-a-half-hour group-based sessions delivered in school settings. However, a program review in 2019 found that the service had limited reach, working with around 50 families per year, had poor outcomes with only one-third of children achieving results of maintaining or reducing their BMI z score, and was expensive and staff intensive to deliver.

The causes of childhood obesity are complex and multifactorial.[62] Tackling childhood obesity requires a whole-systems approach to create an environment that supports families to make healthier choices, accompanied by targeted individual-level interventions for children who are overweight or obese. Work to address the environmental drivers of excess weight is ongoing in Cornwall and will be a crucial focus of the new healthy weight strategy.

---

[61] Wild, C.E., Rawiri, N.T., Willing, E.J., Hofman, P.L. and Anderson, Y.C., 2021. What affects programme engagement for Māori families? A qualitative study of a family-based, multidisciplinary healthy lifestyle programme for children and adolescents. Journal of Paediatrics and Child Health, 57(5), pp.670–676.

[62] Ang, Y.N., Wee, B.S., Poh, B.K. and Ismail, M.N., 2013. Multifactorial influences of childhood obesity. Current Obesity Reports, 2(1), pp.10–22.

Objective

Cornwall Council sought to commission a provider to work closely with their Healthy Cornwall and Public Health groups to lead the development and pilot delivery of a new evidence-informed tier 2 lifestyle weight management program for children aged 5–12 years old in Cornwall. The program will form the basis of a new tier 2 healthy weight offer to children and families and will comprise a key component of the local healthy weight care pathway.

Methods

The project utilized the Method for Program Adaptation through Community Engagement (m-PACE) when tailoring interventions for new populations. This evidenced-based method provides a systematic procedure for obtaining high-quality community feedback and adjudicating recommendations on program developments. The m-PACE method is utilized to uncover local needs through the following:

- Engaging with community members, in particular focusing on areas where inequalities mean that children are more at risk of being overweight and obese

- Collecting parents' and children's feedback through individual interviews

- Conducting focus groups with families after 6 weeks of using the program

Interviews and focus groups are used to understand barriers and facilitators to engagement with healthy weight services and understand local children and families' requirements of a tier 2 lifestyle weight management program. Mixed research methods capture the opinions of more and less vocal community members and reduce the influence of social desirability bias that might otherwise sway data collection. Community members were recruited through multiple channels, including primary care, local media, and offline recruitment in community hubs.

Milestones

The multidisciplinary team broke down the project into the following packages:

- *Month 1*: Stakeholder engagement

    A group of stakeholders will be invited to participate in planning and ongoing monitoring meetings.

- *Months 2–4*: Community engagement

    Community engagement activities will be held, including recruitment of prospective service users. Feedback will be collated into a formal report of findings and recommendations for program development.

- *Months 5–6*: Program development

    The development team used feedback from community engagement to develop the digital and real-world weight management program (syllabus, contents, materials) to ensure suitability for the children and families in Cornwall, resulting in a clinically reviewed program ready for a pilot.

- Months 7–11: Pilot

  Train all staff involved in the delivery of the program.
  Recruit participants to trial the newly developed tier 2
  lifestyle weight management program. A pilot report
  will detail participant engagement, feedback from
  interviews and focus groups, and changes in clinical,
  quality of life, and mental health outcomes.

- Months 11–12: Program modifications and service
  mobilization

  Utilizing post-pilot insight, integrate the tailored tier 2
  lifestyle weight management program into the weight
  management pathways offered across Cornwall.

Evaluation

Feedback from participating children and their families is requested in
the form of structured interviews, surveys using regulatory-compliant
software, and focus groups. Once analyzed, data will be compiled into
a formal report sharing high-quality feedback and recommendations
to decide on program adaptations. Engagement data collected through
attendance, in-platform telemetry, and qualitative feedback, including
structured interviews and focus groups, will be used with quantitative
feedback and clinical outcomes from all participants to inform continuous
improvement.

Impact of the Project

Data shows a higher than expected engagement with socioeconomically
deprived communities with a significant proportion sharing health voice
symptom data (88 percent). Health outcomes are still being analyzed for
publication in a peer-reviewed journal.

Summary

Precision health is a predictive, preventative, personalized, and participative approach to improving individual and population health. A precision approach is already saving lives, giving medical professionals more options, and keeping families healthier for longer. Patients can benefit directly from a precision health approach by having access to their data, tailored behavioral and lifestyle change support, improved adherence to treatments, and real-time monitoring for changes in health. Yet, it will take time to transition from a typical one-size-fits-all strategy to a value-based, personalized, data-driven methodology that focuses on prevention rather than a reaction to advancing disease.

The social and behavioral sciences must collaborate with others to advance precision health research. The net result is anticipated to be a reduction in the overall cost of healthcare. However, research has yet to demonstrate that claim except for a few unique items. Innovators must continue to create evidence to support the claim that precision health can enhance results while minimizing costs. As the case examples in this chapter highlight, the promise of precision medicine in better preventing, predicting, and treating disease is becoming a reality.

Index

A

© Arjun Panesar 2023
A. Panesar, *Precision Health and Artificial Intelligence*,
https://doi.org/10.1007/978-1-4842-9162-7

B

C

D

Printed in the United States
by Baker & Taylor Publisher Services